The Complete Anti-Inflammatory Diet for Beginners

Ultimate Guide to Restoring Your Immune System, Healing Inflammation, and Reversing Disease

EMMA COLLINS

Copyright © 2022 Emma Collins

All rights reserved.
The content contained within this book may not be reproduced, duplicated, or transmitted without direct written permission from the author or the publisher.
Under no circumstances will any blame or legal responsibility be held against the publisher, or author, for any damages, reparation, or monetary loss due to the information contained within this book—either directly or indirectly.

Legal Notice:
This book is copyright protected. This book is only for personal use. You cannot amend, distribute, sell, use, quote, or paraphrase any part of the content within this book without the author or publisher's consent.

Disclaimer Notice:
Please note the information contained within this document is for educational and entertainment purposes only. All effort has been executed to present accurate, up-to-date, and reliable, complete information. No warranties of any kind are declared or implied. Readers acknowledge that the author is not engaging in the rendering of legal, financial, medical, or professional advice. The content within this book has been derived from various sources. Please consult a licensed professional before attempting any techniques outlined in this book. By reading this document, the reader agrees that under no circumstances is the author responsible for any losses, direct or indirect, which are incurred as a result of the use of the information contained within this document, including, but not limited to, — errors, omissions, or inaccuracies.

ISBN: 9798359312974

"Your diet is a bank account. Good food choices are good investments."

~Bethenny Frankel

Table of Contents

Part I: Gluten and Disease 15
    Introduction 17
Chapter One: What is Inflammation? 20
    Inflammation and Chronic Disease 21
    Understanding the Root of Inflammation and Coeliac Disease 22
        The Link Between Inflammation and Obesity 23
        The Bottom Line 24
Chapter Two: Chronic Disease, Pain, and Gluten 25
    What Is Chronic Pain? 26
    The Link Between Chronic Pain and Gluten 27
        Heart Disease and Hypertension 29
    Inflammation and Type-II Diabetes 31
        Chronic Pain and Insomnia 32
    Why Gluten Free? 33
Chapter Three: Allergies and Gluten 35
    How is Inflammation Connected to Allergies? 36
    What is the difference between a food allergy and intolerance? 37
    What are the most common food allergies and intolerances? 39
        Allergies 39

How do I know if I have a food allergy or intolerance?.........40
    What is Histamine?...41
    Identifying Hives 42
Where is histamine found? 44
What does histamine do in the body?..................................44
What are the symptoms of a food allergy or intolerance? 45
    Symptoms..45
    Anaphylaxis 46
    When should one go to the doctor? 46
How is a food allergy or intolerance treated?......................47
Can a food allergy or intolerance be prevented? 47
    Common Symptoms of Food Allergies.............................48
    Triggers for Food Allergies...50
    How to Avoid Triggers 51
    Food Allergies in Adults versus Children..........................52
    Additional Causes and Effects of Excessive and Chronic Release of Histamine..53
    The Immune System, Allergies, and Stress 55
    The Harm of Chronic Use of Anti-Inflammatory Medication 55
    Lists of Common Side Effects of Antihistamine Drugs 56
Chapter Four: Allergies, Infection, and Food.........................57
Infection 58

- Infections Explained Further 59
  - How their effects manifest inside the body 60
  - Infections caused by viruses 61
  - Infections caused by bacteria 63
  - Infections caused by fungi 65
  - Infections caused by bacteria 66
  - Infections caused by prions 67
    - Causes 68
    - Symptoms 69
- Lists of Common Infections 70
  - Common Infections in Children and Young Adults 70
  - Common Infections in Older Adults 71
- Foods that need to be avoided: "Is this Gluten-Free?" 71
- What is a Gluten-Free Diet? 73
- Chapter Five: Processed Foods and Its Dangers 77
- What are Processed Foods? 78
  - Are foods that have been processed unhealthy to eat? 79
  - Added sugar 81
  - Artificial Ingredients 82
  - Refined carbohydrates 83
  - Low in Nutrients 84
  - A diet low in fiber 85
  - Quick calories 86

- Trans fats 86
- Sugar and Inflammation 88
  - The link between sugar and inflammation 88
  - Other ways Sugar can Affect the Body. 90
- Part II: The Heart of the Matter – Gluten-Free Living 93
- Introduction 95
- Chapter Six: Nutritional Necessities 96
  - The Importance of a Balanced Diet in Many Inflammatory Conditions 96
    - Difference between True Hunger and Cravings 99
  - Know How to Keep Track of your Food Intake 100
  - Why Anti-Inflammatory Diets? 101
  - Can a Diet Affect Inflammation? 103
    - When to Expect Results 105
    - Simple guidelines to follow to reduce inflammation through diet 106
  - Anti-Inflammatory Diet Principles 107
- Chapter Seven: The Anti-Inflammation Diet 109
  - Lifestyle Alert: Gluten-Free Protein 109
  - Types of Fats 110
    - Saturated and Unsaturated Fats 111
    - Saturated fats 112
    - Unsaturated fats 113

- Trans Fats 116
  - Are foods without trans fats healthier than other foods? 117
  - Omega-6 Importance 118
    - Uses 120
    - Sources from the Diet 126
  - How you Can Prevent Omega-6 Fats from Promoting Inflammation (Tips) 127
  - Lists of Foods that Help Decrease Inflammation 128
- Chapter Eight: Enhancing the Quality of Mealtimes 131
  - Anti-Inflammatory Cooking: A Gluten-Free (or Low Gluten Diet) 131
  - The Anti-Inflammation Diet in Summary (Gluten-Free Version) 133
  - Fast and Easy Gluten-Free Recipes 136
  - A Seven-Day Meal Plan 136
- Chapter Nine: Foods and Substitution 139
  - Sample Gluten-Free List – Shopping 139
  - What to eliminate, what to substitute, and the directions. 142
  - Modifying Recipes for an Anti-Inflammatory Gluten-Free Diet 145
  - Lists of Items to be kept on Hand Always 147
- Chapter Ten: Anti-inflammation Recipes & Meal Planning 149
  - Sample Anti-Inflammatory Menus for a Week 150

Anti-Inflammatory/Gluten-Free (Dinner) Menus for Four Weeks 152

Chapter Eleven: How to Cook and Prepare Food to Prevent Infection 154

    Temperature control 154

    Purchasing edible products 155

    Getting ready to cook the food 155

    Preventing the food from becoming contaminated while it is being prepared. 156

    Cleaning and sanitizing utensils 157

    Cooking 158

    The process of chilling food 160

    Rewarming the food 161

    Keeping food at a suitable temperature 161

Chapter Twelve: Money-Saving Tips for Preparing your Food 162

    Keep your Recipes Simple 162

    Make Swaps, Narrow It Down, or Leave It Out! 163

    Combine Similar Items 164

    Make Your Meal Meatless 165

    Better to cook at home than eat at a restaurant 166

    Buy in Bulk 167

    Plan Ahead 168

    Utilize your Freezer 169

Chapter Thirteen: What is Better for The Planet When it comes to food consumption 170

    Find out exactly what's in your food. 171

    Start cultivating your garden. 171

    Adopt a diet that is high in plant foods. 172

    Diversify your diet 173

Conclusion 174

Delicious Anti-Inflammation Recipes to Keep Your Family Healthy 176

    Greek white beans in tomato sauce 176

    Spicy corn & black bean salad 179

    Hummus with veggies 181

    Vegetarian chili 182

    Creamy polenta with ratatouille 184

    I pack instant polenta 184

    Baked Oatmeal 186

    Breakfast casserole 188

    Felafel with tahini & tzatziki 190

    Gazpacho 193

    Roasted Garlic Cauliflower Soup 195

    Bean Burger 197

    Frittata with low-fat cheese 199

    Polenta lasagna 201

Shredded part-skim mozzarella cheese............................202

Lentil burger 203

Lentil Meatloaf 205

Broccoli Souffle 208

Veggie Terrines 210

Jamaican Rice and Peas..212

Pomegranate Smoothie..214

Watermelon-Pineapple-Ginger Juice...............................215

Rice with vermicelli...216

Warm Eggplant and Goat Cheese Sandwiches 218

Tomato crostini...220

Lemon and roasted sage chicken 222

Orange and Duck Confit Salad 224

Zucchini Spaghetti..226

Part I: Gluten and Disease

Emma Collins

The Complete Anti-Inflammatory Diet for Beginners

Introduction

Throughout the ride home from school, my 7-year-old was quiet, and yes, I know kids tend to be worn out after school and might even sleep on the ride home, but not my daughter. There was something off. She wasn't looking at me, and she wasn't singing to any of my favorite songs, which were now her favorite songs, and most baffling, she wasn't asking me what I had baked at home.

My probes fell on deaf ears, but my buzzing mind didn't go deaf because she had just changed schools and got forbid she was being bullied. I waited till bedtime, and for some reason, I was nervous about asking her again because I wasn't quite sure how she would react; she wasn't even a 'tweenager' yet. I finally got her to talk, and amidst tears, she told me how she had 'earned' herself a new name, with McBoogers for a suffix.

Yes, she was being bullied for things to which I couldn't find a lasting solution. Her allergies ... I think the word allergy underestimates the serious discomfort and stressful living my poor child was facing. They seemed to be taking over.

Month after month, in every season, she had allergies. We gave out our Maine Coon because we thought she was allergic to cats. Unfortunately, no progress was made, and she still had endless itching, sneezing, runny nose, and just ongoing discomfort. It was messing with her sleep, so we took her to an allergist, and she got put on some medications, but they weren't cures. They helped alleviate her symptoms' gravity, but I wanted her to be free from despair. I want you to take comfort in knowing that you're not alone; whatever type of inflammation you suffer, you're not alone.

When it comes to wanting a better life for our children, we often think of providing them with material things - a safe home, a good education, and plenty of love. But what if there was something more we could do to ensure our children's success and happiness?

According to Dr. Robert Lustig, an expert on childhood obesity and diabetes, one of the most important things we can do for our children is to help them avoid inflammation.

The Complete Anti-Inflammatory Diet for Beginners

Inflammation is at the root of many chronic diseases and allergies, starting early in life. Dr. Lustig believes that half of all American adults currently suffer from inflammation.

So how can we help our children, friends, and family members avoid this fate? Teaching them to eat healthy foods will help reduce inflammation in their bodies. That is the essence of this book. Please keep in mind that I'm not an expert. I'm just a random mother. I devoted tons of hours to reading every possible website, book, blog, or magazine about inflammation. And I also spent long hours chatting with other people, in real life or on social media, to get all the information mentioned in this book. Whatever book I started to read, I found incomplete. There was just partial information, so I decided to write this book to help you, the reader, see all the information in one place. Hopefully, I did it right. If so, I'd be grateful for an honest review of my book.

Thank you.

Emma Collins

Chapter One: What is Inflammation?

Inflammation is the body's natural response to injury or infection. The inflammatory process helps to remove harmful stimuli and begin the healing process. However, inflammation that persists or occurs excessively can lead to various chronic diseases.

There are two types of inflammation: acute and chronic. Acute inflammation is a normal and healthy response typically lasting for a few days. Chronic inflammation, on the other hand, is a prolonged state of low-grade inflammation that can last for months or years. This type of inflammation is linked to several chronic diseases, such as heart disease, cancer, and diabetes.

Inflammation and Chronic Disease

Chronic inflammation is thought to play a role in developing several chronic diseases, such as heart disease, cancer, and diabetes.

Heart Disease

Inflammation is a well-known risk factor for heart disease. One of the earliest signs of heart disease is the presence of inflammation in the arteries. This inflammation is caused by the accumulation of plaque on the artery walls. Plaque is made up of cholesterol, inflammatory cells, and other substances. Over time, plaque can harden and narrow the arteries, leading to reduced blood flow and increased risk of heart attack or stroke.

Cancer

Chronic inflammation has also been linked to cancer. The exact mechanisms are not fully understood, but it is thought that chronic inflammation may promote the growth of cancerous cells or tumors.

Diabetes

Inflammation is also a key factor in the development of type 2 diabetes. In this form of diabetes, the body's cells become resistant to insulin, a hormone that helps to regulate blood sugar levels. This resistance leads to high blood sugar levels, which can damage different organs in the body over time.

Understanding the Root of Inflammation and Coeliac Disease

When discussing inflammation, it is important to understand the root cause. In many cases, chronic inflammation is caused by autoimmune diseases. Autoimmune diseases occur when the body's immune system mistakenly attacks healthy cells and tissues. One of the most well-known autoimmune diseases is coeliac disease.

Coeliac disease is a condition that damages the lining of the small intestine and prevents it from absorbing nutrients properly. This damage is caused by an immune reaction to gluten, a protein found in wheat, barley, and rye. When someone with coeliac disease eats foods containing gluten, their immune system attacks the lining of the small intestine. This damaged villus makes it difficult for the body to absorb nutrients, leading to various health problems.

The Complete Anti-Inflammatory Diet for Beginners

Coeliac disease affects 1 in 100 people worldwide. It is estimated that 83% of people with coeliac disease are undiagnosed or misdiagnosed. Many people with the coeliac disease experience no symptoms or only mild symptoms that can be easily mistaken for something else. For this reason, getting tested for coeliac disease is important if you have a family member with the condition or if you're experiencing any unexplained gastrointestinal issues.

If you have been diagnosed with coeliac disease, the only treatment is to follow a strict gluten-free diet. This means avoiding all foods that contain wheat, barley, and rye. While this may seem like a daunting task, there are many delicious and gluten-free foods available. You can easily create nutritious and satisfying meals with a little creativity and effort.

The Link Between Inflammation and Obesity

Obesity is another common cause of chronic inflammation. Obesity is a body mass index (BMI) of 30 or above. BMI is a measure of body fat based on height and weight. People who are obese often have higher levels of inflammatory markers in their blood, even if they don't have any other health problems.

The link between obesity and inflammation is thought to be due to the release of pro-inflammatory substances from fat cells. These substances can damage different organs in the body and lead to chronic inflammation.

Weight loss is the most effective way to reduce inflammation caused by obesity. Even a small amount of weight loss can significantly impact inflammation levels. If you struggle to lose weight, speak to your doctor or a registered dietitian. They can create a weight loss plan tailored to your individual needs and goals.

The Bottom Line

Inflammation is a key factor in the development of many chronic diseases. Understanding the root cause of inflammation is essential for preventing and treating these conditions. Coeliac disease, obesity, and other autoimmune diseases are common causes of chronic inflammation. If you have been diagnosed with one of these conditions, following a strict gluten-free diet or losing weight can help to reduce inflammation and improve your overall health.

Chapter Two: Chronic Disease, Pain, and Gluten

Chronic disease is a condition that persists for a long time. Many chronic diseases are the result of inflammation. Inflammation is the body's natural response to injury or infection. While acute inflammation is a short-term response that helps to heal the body, chronic inflammation can last for months or even years.

Chronic inflammation is linked to many health conditions, including heart disease, cancer, and Alzheimer's. In some cases, chronic inflammation can lead to chronic pain.

Emma Collins

What Is Chronic Pain?

Chronic pain is defined as pain that lasts for more than 12 weeks. It can be caused by an injury, illness, or underlying health condition. Chronic pain can be mild, moderate, or severe. It can also vary in frequency and intensity.

Chronic pain can have a major impact on your quality of life. It can interfere with your ability to work, sleep, and participate in activities you enjoy. Chronic pain can also lead to depression and anxiety.

There are many different types of chronic pain. The most common types include:

- Headaches

- Arthritis pain

- Back pain

- Cancer pain

- Nerve pain

- Fibromyalgia

Treating chronic pain can be difficult. There is no one-size-fits-all approach. Treatment depends on the underlying cause of the pain and the severity of the symptoms. Pain medications, physical therapy, and lifestyle changes are often used to treat chronic pain.

The Link Between Chronic Pain and Gluten

There is growing evidence linking gluten to chronic pain. Gluten is a protein found in wheat, barley, and rye. It can also be found in some processed foods and medications.

People with celiac disease are sensitive to gluten. When they eat gluten, their immune system reacts by damaging the lining of the small intestine. This can lead to inflammation and other health problems.

Non-celiac gluten sensitivity (NCGS) is another condition linked to gluten intolerance. People with NCGS don't have celiac disease but experience symptoms after eating gluten.

The symptoms of NCGS are similar to those of celiac disease, but they're less severe. They can include abdominal pain, bloating, diarrhea, fatigue, and headaches.

NCGS is often difficult to diagnose because the symptoms are similar to those of other conditions. No blood test or biopsy can confirm the diagnosis. The only way to know if you have NCGS is to eliminate gluten from your diet and see if your symptoms improve.

A growing body of research suggests that NCGS is a real condition affecting many people. It's estimated that up to 6% of the population has NCGS.

Researchers are still trying to understand the exact link between gluten and chronic pain. Gluten-sensitive individuals may have a heightened inflammatory response to the protein. This could lead to inflammation in the nervous system, leading to pain.

There is also evidence that gluten may cause changes in the gut microbiome, which can lead to inflammation and pain. The gut microbiome is the collection of bacteria in the digestive tract. These bacteria play an important role in gut health and immunity.

A study about the effect of a gluten-free diet on gut microbiota composition in patients with celiac disease and non-celiac gluten/wheat sensitivity published in 2015 found that people with NCGS had a different composition of gut bacteria than those without the condition. The study found that people with NCGS had lower levels of helpful bacteria, including Lactobacillus and Bifidobacterium.

Another study found that a gluten-free diet improved symptoms in people with NCGS. The study participants who followed a gluten-free diet for six weeks significantly reduced abdominal pain, bloating, and fatigue. They also had an increase in beneficial gut bacteria.

Heart Disease and Hypertension

Gluten is also linked to heart disease and hypertension.

Heart disease is the leading cause of death in the United States. It's estimated that one in four deaths in the country is caused by heart disease.

Hypertension, or high blood pressure, is a major risk factor for heart disease. It's estimated that 66% of people with hypertension will develop heart disease.

Researchers believe that gluten may contribute to heart disease and hypertension by causing inflammation. Now the question is, how does inflammation cause heart disease and hypertension?

Some researchers believe that inflammation caused by gluten can damage the lining of the arteries. This damage can lead to the buildup of plaque, which can narrow or block the arteries.

Inflammation can also cause high blood pressure by affecting the function of the endothelium. The endothelium is the inner lining of blood vessels. It helps regulate blood pressure by relaxing and constricting the arteries.

If the endothelium is damaged, it doesn't work as well. This can cause the arteries to constrict, leading to high blood pressure.

A 2013 study about the evaluation of endothelial functions in patients with celiac disease found that a gluten-free diet improved endothelial function in people with celiac disease. The study participants who followed a gluten-free diet for one year significantly improved endothelial function.

The researchers believe the gluten-free diet may have improved endothelial function by reducing inflammation.

Inflammation and Type-II Diabetes

Type-II diabetes is a condition that occurs when the body becomes resistant to insulin. Insulin is a hormone that helps regulate blood sugar levels.

When the body doesn't respond properly to insulin, blood sugar levels can become too high. Over time, this can damage the pancreas, nerves, and blood vessels.

Type-II diabetes is a serious condition that can lead to complications such as heart disease, stroke, and kidney damage.

It's estimated that 34% of people with type-II diabetes die from heart disease.

Gluten has been linked to inflammation and an increased risk of type-II diabetes.

A 2010 study found that people with celiac disease had a nearly four-fold increased risk of type-II diabetes.

Another study found that a gluten-free diet improved blood sugar control in people with type-II diabetes. The study participants who followed a gluten-free diet

Chronic Pain and Insomnia

Inflammation can contribute to numerous types of chronic pain, including fibromyalgia. Inflammation may be a symptom of fibromyalgia, even though the condition is not considered an inflammatory disease. Fibromyalgia is characterized by widespread pain and widespread muscle and joint pain. Sleep habits that are frequently interrupted are one factor that contributes to the length of time it takes for fibromyalgia patients to feel better. It is well known that our immune system is active twenty-four hours a day, seven days a week, cleaning out our bodies and creating repairs, especially while we are asleep. This cleansing and repair process cannot function at an ideal level if sleep is disrupted, which is the case for many fibromyalgia patients.

The Complete Anti-Inflammatory Diet for Beginners

Why Gluten Free?

Because of the lack of proper cleaning within the system, cells, and tissues affected by this impairment of the process of cleaning and repairing suffer from inflammation that lasts longer. The accumulation of waste items starts right away. Serotonin levels are disrupted in many persons who struggle with this disorder. This fluctuation in level can severely affect a person's mood, ability to sleep, creation of new tissue, and metabolism of carbohydrates, all of which are important for sustained energy levels throughout the day. People who suffer from fibromyalgia need to have a functioning digestive system. A diet that is nutritious and does not contain gluten may be able to break this negative cycle and assist in reducing the unpleasant gluten symptoms of the sickness by assisting in the reduction of inflammation. Inflammation is minimized, and serotonin releases are improved when the gastrointestinal system functions properly. This can improve a person's mood and make it easier for them to get a decent sleep.

The recovery of the immune system's capacity to rid the body of waste and repair damage as you sleep is a welcome benefit of this treatment. Gluten-free diets are becoming increasingly popular as a viable treatment option for various health conditions, including chronic pain and insomnia. Gluten is a composite of plant proteins that can be found in a wide variety of grains and other foods. Gluten-free diets exclude all sorts of food with a significant level of gluten in their composition.

Curiously, rice and corn both contain gluten, but in a form that does not provoke symptoms of celiac disease, and as a result, both foods are believed to be gluten-free. In addition, gluten is present in some form or another in all cereals.

Chapter Three: Allergies and Gluten

In most cases, allergies result from the immune system's overreaction to the presence of foreign chemicals. A strong immune system is prepared to defend the body against introducing any foreign substance into your system if it comes into contact with it. When functioning properly, the immune system guards the body against harmful pathogens, including infections and diseases. On the other hand, the immune system tends to overreact since it cannot always tell the difference between beneficial, neutral, and dangerous intruders. This hyperactive immunity can cause your body to go into a tailspin, reacting with prolonged inflammation to even 'Harmless Visitors,' which can cause further harm. Allergens are the names of these "Visitors" that cause allergic reactions. The inflammation that results can come on suddenly or linger for a long time, creating allergic reactions ranging from moderate to severe.

Emma Collins

How is Inflammation Connected to Allergies?

Allergies are a reaction of the immune system to a foreign substance, such as pollen, pet dander, or dust mites. In most cases, allergies are not harmful. However, they can cause uncomfortable symptoms, such as sneezing, itching, and swelling.

Allergies occur when the immune system overreacts to a foreign substance. The immune system produces antibodies to "attack" the foreign substance. This release of antibodies causes the symptoms of an allergy.

The link between inflammation and allergies has been well-established. Inflammation is a response of the immune system to infection or injury.

An immune system overreaction causes allergies and autoimmune diseases. In both cases, the immune system attacks healthy tissue.

Inflammation is a key component of the allergic response. The release of inflammatory chemicals causes the symptoms of an allergy.

In some cases, inflammation can lead to chronic allergies. Chronic allergies are a type of allergy that lasts for an extended time. They can cause severe symptoms and be difficult to treat.

Chronic inflammation has been linked to the development of allergies.

The association of celiac disease and allergic disease in a general adult population study found that people with celiac disease had a higher risk of developing allergies. The study participants who followed a gluten-free diet for one year significantly reduced their risk of developing allergies.

The researchers believe the gluten-free diet may have reduced the risk of allergies by reducing inflammation.

What is the difference between a food allergy and intolerance?

Most people who experience adverse reactions to particular foods do so due to a food intolerance rather than an actual food allergy. People frequently get the two conditions mixed up because the signs and symptoms of food intolerance can be very similar to those of a food allergy.

A genuine allergy to food will affect the immune system. Even in very small amounts, the food that causes an allergic reaction can cause a wide variety of symptoms, some of which can be very serious or even life-threatening. On the other hand, symptoms caused by food intolerance are often limited to the digestive tract and are generally less severe.

If you have a food intolerance, you might be able to consume moderate amounts of the food that triggers your reaction without any adverse effects. You could also be able to stop a reaction from happening. If you have trouble digesting lactose, for instance, you might be able to improve your digestion by drinking milk that does not contain lactose or by using lactase enzyme pills like Lactaid.

Some of the following can lead to food intolerance:

Lack of an enzyme, which is required for the complete digestion of food. The inability to digest lactose is a typical case.

Syndrome of the irritable bowel. This long-term disease can result in cramps, as well as both diarrhea and constipation.

Intolerance of many food additives. People prone to asthma attacks because they are sensitive to food additives may find those sulfites, which are used to preserve dried fruit, canned products, and wine, cause their symptoms.

What are the most common food allergies and intolerances?

- Peanuts
- Tree nuts (such as walnuts, pecans, and almonds)
- Fish
- Shellfish
- Milk
- Eggs
- Soy
- Wheat

Allergies

- Symptoms such as bloating, cramping, or gas
- Heartburn
- Headaches
- Irritability or anxiousness may also be present.

An allergic reaction to food occurs when the body's immune system confuses a food component for a threat and launches an attack against it. It can affect your entire body, not just your stomach. Among the possible symptoms are:

- Rashes, hives, or skin that is extremely itchy
- Uneasy and shallow breaths
- Chest pain

How do I know if I have a food allergy or intolerance?

It's not always easy to distinguish between a food allergy and intolerance. Both can cause similar symptoms, but they are quite different. Here's a look at the key differences between the two:

A food allergy occurs when your body has an adverse reaction to a particular food or ingredient. This is usually due to the immune system response, which can be severe. On the other hand, intolerance is when your body has difficulty digesting a certain food. This is often due to a lack of enzymes that help break down the food.

The Complete Anti-Inflammatory Diet for Beginners

A food allergy can include hives, swelling, difficulty breathing, and anaphylaxis. Intolerance symptoms are usually less severe and may include bloating, gas, diarrhea, and nausea.

When we start a new diet or lifestyle, we may experience increased gas and bloating. This is because our bodies are adjusting to the new foods we eat and the change in our routine. For some people, this gas and bloating are due to food intolerances.

There are many types of food intolerances, but the most common ones include lactose intolerance and gluten intolerance. If you suspect a food intolerance, you must speak with your doctor or a registered dietitian to find out for sure. They can help you identify which foods you should avoid and how to create a healthy, balanced diet that meets your needs.

What is Histamine?

The body produces antibodies in response to exposure to allergens to defend against potential threats. In response, many antibodies attach themselves to the surface of the cells that comprise tissue within the body. They are patiently waiting for the next assault by the allergen identified as a potential hazard to the body. They collect a variety of substances from the blood as it travels through the system as they are on guard, which ultimately leads to inflammation. When there is a further attack, the allergen is re-adhered to by certain antibodies, which then causes the release of a chemical. Histamine is one of these carefully engineered molecules, and it plays a role in the allergic response that the body sets up.

Histamine is responsible for many uncomfortable symptoms connected with allergic reactions, such as sneezing, runny noses, itching, and many more. Anti-allergy drugs are also known as antihistamines, and their primary function is to block the ability of histamines to bind to their respective receptors. There are two stages to an allergic reaction. The chemicals are released shortly after exposure to an allergen, which is the early phase. After several hours since the first exposure, a late-phase reaction can develop when inflammatory cells are called in as backup. Hives are a common skin symptom brought on by allergic reactions. Hives can appear anywhere on the body, although most commonly appear on the arms, legs, and chest. However, they can also appear in other regions of the body. Mouth, tongue, and throat swelling can result from a severe allergic reaction.

Identifying Hives

Hives manifest themselves on the skin's surface in their most common form as elevated, ruddy lumps (welts). Itching and general discomfort, such as stinging or burning, are frequently present alongside the condition. They can be as small as an inch or as large as a small dish. Their dimensions are quite variable. It's possible that the entire affected area of the skin could swell up and become irritated. The lips may swell up, and the skin around your eyes might also swell up.

As was just discussed, hives can arise suddenly or gradually over time. Even though welts are rather prevalent, it is not always the case that they indicate an allergic reaction. When hives do form on a person, they often begin on one area of the body and then swiftly spread to other places of the body when they occur. It is not unheard of for the welts to swell up and combine with other hives as time passes (or welts). On rare occasions, these papules and pustules can grow to cover significant areas of the skin. It is possible for the hives to spread, which can result in uncomfortable feelings such as shivering, burning, and acute itching. The welts may form, fade, and then resurface a few minutes, a few days, or even several weeks later. Allergic reactions to a wide variety of allergens, including those connected with food allergies, can cause hives on the skin.

Emma Collins

Where is histamine found?

In human beings, histamine may be found in almost all of the body's tissues, predominantly stored in the granules of the mast cells that make up these tissues. Granules carrying histamine are also seen inside basophils, a type of blood cell.

What does histamine do in the body?

They are chemicals that are produced by your immune system. Histamines perform the role of doormen at a club. They assist your body in getting rid of whatever is causing you discomfort, which in this situation is an allergy trigger, also known as an "allergen." Histamines kick off the process that gets allergens out of your body or off your skin and into the environment.

What are the symptoms of a food allergy or intolerance?

Symptoms

An allergic reaction to a specific food may only be somewhat bothersome rather than life-threatening for some individuals. An allergic reaction to food can be a terrifying experience; in some cases, it can even be life-threatening. Meal allergy symptoms typically manifest from a few minutes to two hours after consuming the allergenic food. Sometimes the onset of symptoms can be delayed by several hours.

The following are some of the most prevalent indications and symptoms of food allergies:

- Tingling or stinging sensations in the oral cavity
- Itchy rashes, eczema, and hives
- The lips, face, tongue, neck, and other body regions, may swell up.
- Symptoms such as wheezing, stuffy nose, and difficulty breathing
- Abdominal pain, diarrhea, nausea, or vomiting
- symptoms such as vertigo, lightheadedness, or fainting

Emma Collins

Anaphylaxis

Food allergies can potentially bring on a life-threatening allergic reaction known as anaphylaxis in certain individuals. This can create signs and symptoms that are potentially life-threatening, including:

- The narrowing and constriction of the airways are symptoms.
- A sore throat or the feeling of having something caught in your throat might make it difficult to breathe.
- A precipitous drop in blood pressure characterizes shock
- Rapid pulse
- Lightheadedness, dizziness, or even loss of consciousness may occur.
- Treatment in an emergency setting is necessary for anaphylaxis. If the anaphylaxis is not addressed, it can lead to a coma or possibly death.

When should one go to the doctor?

If you experience symptoms of a food allergy soon after eating, you should consult your primary care physician or an allergist. Visit your healthcare practitioner as soon as you notice symptoms of an allergic reaction, if at all feasible. Your healthcare provider will be better able to diagnose you due to this.

How is a food allergy or intolerance treated?

If you think you might have a food allergy, you should stay away from the food in question until you have an appointment with your doctor. If you consume the meal and experience a moderate response, taking available over-the-counter antihistamines may help relieve your symptoms. If your reaction is more severe or you experience any signs or symptoms of anaphylaxis, you should seek immediate medical attention.

Can a food allergy or intolerance be prevented?

The only method to protect yourself from an allergic reaction to food is to steer clear of the offending item and anything else that might include it as an ingredient. Although food intolerance and food allergies may overlap symptoms like diarrhea and stomach pain, food intolerance does not activate the immune system, does not pose a life-threatening risk and is not the same as a food allergy.

Common Symptoms of Food Allergies

Itchy hives are only one of the many outward manifestations that can accompany a food allergy. As a result of my investigation, I've discovered that particular meals have the potential to bring on a wide range of health issues. As we have shown previously, there is a connection between inflammation and some illnesses, diseases, and food allergies, most of which are associated with gluten. One of the most common of these is celiac disease. As we have recently discovered, an allergic reaction can be triggered by various chemicals. The direct relationship between particular foods, specifically those containing gluten (the protein found in wheat), and food allergies are what I found to be the most startling and disturbing! Because gluten and milk are the triggers for two of the most frequent types of food allergies, it is essential to realize the benefits of a gluten and dairy-free diet. Permit me to go into further detail.

The reaction of the immune system to certain proteins that are present in food is what causes an allergic reaction to food. Certain meals, similar to other triggers of allergic reactions, have the potential to stimulate the body to release histamine. A wide range of symptoms, including runny nose, sneezing, hives, stomach cramps, diarrhea, and even anaphylaxis, are possible outcomes of this illness (an extremely serious condition that occurs rapidly and occasionally, resulting in death). And if that isn't worrying enough, consider that this response can occur anytime. A mild to severe reaction is possible for everyone allergic (as my daughter did). Some antibodies may become activated when the offending food is taken, interacting with the food particles and causing an autoimmune-inflammatory response. Inflammation, as we now know, can impede the capacity of the body to heal itself and correctly metabolize the food it eats.

In addition, these food allergens are typically not digested correctly, which causes them to accumulate in the liver, kidneys, and other organs responsible for detoxifying the body. After removing gluten from their diet, many individuals discover that they no longer have allergic reactions to the foods they eat. Among the common symptoms are those that we have already singled out. The following graphic overview shows the many indications and symptoms of food allergies.

The signs and symptoms of a food allergy can range from quite minor to extremely severe. They may manifest themselves immediately or up to two hours after consuming the offending dish.

Mild symptoms include:

- Itching or tingling in the mouth
- Hives, rash, or redness on the skin
- Nausea, stomach cramps, diarrhea, or vomiting

Severe symptoms include:

- Tightening of the throat
- Difficulty breathing
- Drop in blood pressure
- Loss of consciousness

You should see a doctor if you have these symptoms after eating. You may be experiencing anaphylaxis, a life-threatening reaction.

Triggers for Food Allergies

Many things can trigger a food allergy. The most common triggers are:

- Certain foods: Milk, eggs, peanuts, tree nuts, soy, wheat, fish, and shellfish are the most common offenders.

- Medications: Some antibiotics and NSAIDs can cause allergies.

- Insect stings: People allergic to bee stings may also be allergic to insects, such as wasps or hornets.

- Latex: People with latex allergies may also be allergic to certain fruits and vegetables.

How to Avoid Triggers

- The best way to avoid an allergic reaction is to avoid the trigger. If you have a food allergy, you must avoid the offending food.

- If you have a latex allergy, you must avoid products containing latex. These include gloves, balloons, and rubber bands.

- If you are allergic to bee stings, you should carry an EpiPen. This is a device that injects a shot of epinephrine, which can stop a severe reaction.

Emma Collins

Food Allergies in Adults versus Children

It's possible that prenatal exposure to allergens or genetics played a role in the development of food sensitivities in infants and young children. If a child is given infant formula rather than breast milk or solid baby food too soon, this might cause damage to the intestinal cells, leading to allergies. This injury frequently occurs when the intestines are not yet developed enough to deal with consumed meals. If a person develops a food allergy later in life, the allergy is typically the result of chemical or physical damage within the intestines' cells. This damage can occur at any point in a person's life. For instance, food poisoning can cause irreversible damage to the gut lining if the toxins produced are not processed and cleared correctly. An autoimmune reaction may be triggered when anything like this occurs, resulting in inflammation in the intestines and the rest of the body. The most damage is typically done to the most delicate regions of the body. When damage develops gradually over time, inflammation can develop, which causes tissue and organ damage. This can lead to an imbalance that lasts for a long period.

Because of this, the first step in mending the damage to tissues and organs is to pay attention to the food one consumes and ensure correct digestion. Altering one's diet and emphasizing easily digested foods is one of the most common and effective ways to alleviate symptoms of a wide range of serious health conditions, including allergies, arthritis, heart disease, skin problems, and asthma discussed earlier. The greater the duration of an allergic reaction to food, the more severe the subsequent harm. To protect your family from getting sick, being diagnosed with a disease, developing an allergy, or being exposed to an infection, the most effective preventative measure is to conduct a thorough investigation into the likelihood that members of your family suffer from gluten intolerance or food allergies.

Additional Causes and Effects of Excessive and Chronic Release of Histamine

Histamine is a molecule always present in our bodies, as we know from the prior discussion. It is produced and stored within cells that are specialized for the purpose, and it assists the immune system in protecting the body against invading organisms and undesirable substances. In addition to these functions, histamine is also one of the "messengers" released by the brain. It assists in the production of gastric acid, which is necessary for digestion within the stomach. According to the research findings, a significant portion of the population is hypersensitive.

Due to this hypersensitivity, large histamine levels may be produced when exposed to environmental allergens or when foods containing allergens are ingested. Histamine levels that are too high might result in various uncomfortable feelings and symptoms, ranging from minor annoyances to severe allergic reactions. Itching on one side of the body may be triggered by high amounts of the chemical histamine. The itching results from additional forms of inflammation and irritation triggered when abnormally high histamine levels are present.

In a similar vein, excessive quantities of histamine can lead to symptoms such as watery, itchy, red eyes, nasal congestion, runny noses, sneezing, irritation of the eyes and ears, and post-nasal drip. In most cases, this kind of reaction is brought on by allergens that are carried via the air. It is also possible for asthmatic reactions to take place when there is an excessive amount of histamine present in the bloodstream. This ailment, which can be quite dangerous and last for a long time, manifests itself when increased mucous discharge from the respiratory system. The most common symptoms include wheezing, trouble breathing, and a tight feeling in the chest. The overproduction of histamines can result in swelling in deep tissue, leading to enlargement of the digestive tract, throat, and mouth and limited breathing, which can be fatal in extreme cases. Anaphylaxis is a condition that can be brought on by a particularly severe reaction to high quantities of histamine. This potentially fatal disorder can manifest in various ways, including a sudden drop in blood pressure, abdominal pain, diarrhea, bloated and inflamed skin, nausea, vomiting, nasal congestion, coughing, wheezing, difficulty breathing, dizziness, and fainting.

The Complete Anti-Inflammatory Diet for Beginners

The Immune System, Allergies, and Stress

Stress's impact on our bodies can result in various unfavorable responses. The capacity to deal with stress is already ingrained in our systems. Stimulating the stress hormone cortisol, which is caused by stress, results in an abrupt increase in one's energy level. Because we live in an extremely stressful society, this response can be activated anytime, even in rush hour traffic. The rapid surge of energy makes it possible for us to either "fight or flee," but the vast majority of the time, we are not in a position to put this additional strength to use. Because there is no mechanism to utilize the sugar in our blood, we frequently end up with consistently high cortisol levels. This sustained spike can have a detrimental effect on one's immune system, increasing the chance of allergic reactions and inflammation and the danger of various health problems associated with stress.

The Harm of Chronic Use of Anti-Inflammatory Medication

When used excessively, any anti-inflammatory medicine carries the potential for certain adverse effects. When it comes to anti-inflammatories, the potential side effects include but are not limited to cardiovascular problems, erectile dysfunction, gastrointestinal problems, inflammatory bowel disease, renal difficulties, difficulties during pregnancy, and difficulties with possible drug interactions. These are just some of the potential side effects! The adverse effects have been made significantly worse due to the increased consumption of anti-inflammatory drugs. Damage to the gastrointestinal tract and the kidneys is the most common adverse response. Ulcers, bleeding in the gastrointestinal tract, and even the possibility of death are all potential adverse effects.

Lists of Common Side Effects of Antihistamine Drugs

There are several side effects related to antihistamine drugs. Some of these side effects are listed below.

- Anxiety

- Drowsiness

- Dry Mouth

- Heart Palpitations Problems

- Constipation Problems

- Urination

Chapter Four: Allergies, Infection, and Food

As can be seen, a distinct pattern is starting to take shape. To maintain our lives, each of our organs must cooperate. The digestive system's job is to break down the food we eat so that it can provide us with energy and keep us in the best possible health. Following digestion, the food is broken down, the nutrients are assimilated into our system, and the waste products are expelled. The more wisely you select your meals, the more efficiently and profitably you will achieve your goals!

Because of this, maintaining a diet that is nutritionally sound and well-balanced can assist us in avoiding many of the health issues that have been addressed this far, as well as the accumulation of waste in the digestive tract. Consuming nutritious foods can assist boost one's energy levels and overall well-being. In addition to the foods we eat, we are continuously subjected to the toxins in our environment. Growth hormones and trace levels of antibiotics, pesticides, and other chemicals can be found in our food, and we unintentionally consume them. Our body's digestive system makes an extra effort to rid itself of harmful substances while processing helpful nutrients. The kidneys and liver collaborate to process the food and drink that we take in. This method, despite its great degree of efficacy, will never produce perfect results. Every one of us distinctly processes food and reacts differently depending on the surrounding environment. Becoming knowledgeable and attuning yourself to your unique requirements is the most efficient method for achieving a good balance in your life. You won't only have an improved appearance and sense of well-being, but you'll also probably have a great deal more energy and a larger capacity to ward off illness and infection.

Infection

As we know, being allergic to something and having bad health strains our systems. Infection is another condition that brings about a decline in immune function. Even if we take every precaution to protect ourselves from outside sources of infection, we will always have viruses, parasites, and yeasts inside our bodies. Even if they are present, there is no reason to assume they will cause harm. On the other hand, when our immune systems are suppressed, we are far more prone to getting sick. When we get sick, our natural tendency is to reach for an antibiotic as our first line of defense against the illness. Antibiotics are not always the best course of treatment, although they sometimes serve a practical purpose. Antibiotics may eliminate pathogenic bacteria, but they also eliminate the helpful bacteria that are naturally present in our bodies, which cause damage to the gut tissue. Extensive research demonstrates a significant link between inflammation, disease, and infection, particularly in conditions associated with the digestive system.

Infections Explained Further

The nature of the pathogen determines how an illness is transmitted as well as the consequences it has on the human body.

The immune system functions as a formidable defense mechanism against infectious pathogens. Despite this, it is possible for pathogens to occasionally overwhelm the immune system's capacity to fight them off. When it reaches this point, an infection is already dangerous.

Some diseases don't cause much of an effect at all. Some of these organisms create poisons or inflammatory compounds that cause the body to react unfavorably. Because of this diversity, some infections are light, and you may not even notice them, while others might be serious and threaten your life. Some infectious agents cannot be treated.

There are several different vectors through which infection might propagate.

Many distinct pathogens exist, including bacteria, viruses, fungi, and parasites. They differ in several ways, including the following:

- Dimensions
- Shapes
- Functions
- Genetic components

How their effects manifest inside the body

To give just one example, bacteria are far larger than viruses. They invade the host and take over the cells, in contrast to bacteria which may live independently of a host.

The Complete Anti-Inflammatory Diet for Beginners

The treatment will be tailored to address the underlying cause of the infection. The most prevalent and potentially lethal forms of infection are bacteria, viruses, fungi, and prions.

Infections caused by viruses

Infections caused by viruses begin when a person contracts a virus themselves. There may be millions of distinct viruses worldwide, but scientists have only cataloged around 5,000 of them so far. Viruses have a protective coat of protein and lipid (fat) molecules. This coat encases a small portion of the genetic information that the virus carries.

A virus takes over a host, and the virus then attaches itself to a cell. Their genetic material is immediately released when they reach the cell. This substance compels the cell to duplicate the virus, which then causes the virus to proliferate. When the cell dies, it releases new viruses, infecting other cells when they have been created.

However, not all viruses cause their host cell to be destroyed. Some of them can alter the function of the cell. Cancer can be caused by many viruses, including the human papillomavirus (HPV) and the Epstein-Barr virus (EBV). These viruses cause cells to multiply in an uncontrolled manner, which can lead to cancer.

There are some age groups that a virus may specifically target, such as newborns or early children.

Viruses can hibernate for a while before resuming their multiplication. The infected individual may feel healed, yet they risk becoming ill once more if the virus becomes active again.

Infections caused by viruses can include:

The common cold, which is caused by rhinoviruses, coronaviruses, and adenoviruses; encephalitis and meningitis, which are caused by enteroviruses and the herpes simplex virus (HSV); warts and skin infections, which HPV and HSV cause; gastroenteritis, which is caused by norovirus; COVID-19, a respiratory disease that develops after a novel coronavirus infection;

Medication that targets certain viruses can alleviate the symptoms of that virus while it is still present in the body. Either they can stop the virus from reproducing in the host or increase the host's immune system to combat the virus's consequences.

Antibiotics are ineffective against viruses and cannot treat viral infections. These medications will not stop the infection, and using them raises the risk that the virus will become resistant to antibiotics.

The majority of treatments focus on symptom relief so that the immune system can do its job of fighting the virus without any help from medicines.

Infections caused by bacteria

Bacteria are a prokaryote type, another name for single-celled microorganisms.

According to the scientific community, there must be at least one nonillion different microorganisms on Earth. A nonillion is a number composed of a 1 followed by 30 zeros. Bacteria make up a significant portion of the earth's total biomass.

There are three primary forms that bacteria can take:

These are called cocci, and they have a spherical shape.
Bacilli are defined by their rod-like shapes and bear the name.
Spirilla: Spiral bacteria are also known as coiled bacteria. When the coil of a spirillum is wound extremely tightly, the scientific community refers to it as a spirochete.

Bacteria can survive in any environment, from extremely hot to extremely cold temperatures, and some bacteria can even thrive in radioactive waste.

Emma Collins

There are trillions of different strains of bacteria, yet very few of them are responsible for diseases that affect people. Some can dwell harmlessly inside the human body, such as in the gastrointestinal tract or the airways.

Some "good" bacteria seek out and destroy disease-causing bacteria, preventing illness from being caused by the latter. However, some bacterial illnesses can be fatal.

These are the following:

- Cholera
- Diphtheria
- Dysentery
- Plague of bubonic origin
- Tuberculosis
- Typhoid / styphus

The following are some examples of infections caused by bacteria:

- Bacteria cause meningitis
- Middle ear infection
- Pneumonia
- Infection of the upper respiratory tract caused by tuberculosis (although this is usually viral)

- Inflammation of the stomach, food poisoning
- Diseases of the eyes
- Sinusitis (again, more often viral)
- Infections of the urinary tract (UTIs)
- Infections of the skin
- Illnesses that are transferred by sexual contact (STIs)

Antibiotics are medications a doctor can prescribe to treat bacterial infections. However, certain strains can develop resistance to the therapy and continue to thrive despite it.

Infections caused by fungi

Fungi are often multicellular parasites that use enzymes to break down organic stuff and absorb it into their bodies. Yeasts, on the other hand, are a form of organism that only has a single cell.

Reproduction in fungi nearly always occurs through the dissemination of spores, which are single-celled offspring. Fungi often have elongated bodies that are cylindrical and are composed of several tiny filaments that branch off of the primary body.

Fungi can be classified into around 5.1 million different species.

Emma Collins

The upper layers of the skin are home to the development of many fungal diseases, but some of these infections can spread to the deeper layers. When yeast or mold spores are breathed in, a person may develop a fungal illness, such as pneumonia, or an infection that affects the entire body. Systemic infections are another name for these types of illnesses.

Infections caused by bacteria

The human body normally has a population of beneficial bacteria that contribute to the upkeep of the delicate microbial balance. These cover the inside of the intestines, mouth, and vagina, in addition to other anatomical parts.

People who fall into any of the following categories have an increased likelihood of having a fungal infection:

- People who use antibiotics over an extended period.
- They have a compromised immune system due to conditions such as living with HIV or diabetes or receiving chemotherapy treatment. They have undergone a transplant and are taking drugs to keep their body from rejecting the new organ.

Infections caused by fungi include the following:

Diseases include valley fever, coccidioidomycosis, histoplasmosis, candidiasis, athlete's foot, ringworm, and some eye infections.

Infections caused by prions

Prion is the name given to a class of proteins devoid of any genetic content and not often harmful. Prion particles are not considered to be living microbes by the scientific community. On the other hand, if a prion folds into an irregular shape, it has the potential to turn into a rogue agent and induce infection.

The structure of the brain or other components of the nervous system may be altered when prions are present. They are unable to reproduce and do not feed off of the host. Instead, they cause the cells and proteins in the body to behave in an aberrant manner.

Prions are the causative agent in all forms of neurodegenerative disease, all of which are extremely rare but make rapid progress and are ultimately fatal. Creutzfeldt-Jakob disease and bovine spongiform encephalopathy (BSE), more commonly known as mad cow disease, fall into this category (CJD).

Researchers have also shown a connection between Alzheimer's disease and prion infection in certain patients.

In conclusion, ectoparasites such as mites, ticks, lice, and fleas are all capable of causing infections by attaching themselves to the skin or burrowing into it. Ectoparasites can also be blood-sucking arthropods like mosquitoes, which spread disease by feeding on human blood and are sometimes referred to as "bloodsuckers."

Causes

The entry of any kind of organism into the body might be considered the root cause of an illness. An infection caused by a virus, for instance, will be caused by a particular virus.

The symptoms of an infection, such as swelling or a runny nose, are caused by the immune system's attempt to eliminate the foreign organism that has invaded the body to restore health.

When white blood cells rush to the site of an injury to fight off foreign microorganisms, this might lead to a wound becoming filled with pus.

Symptoms

The symptoms of infection vary widely depending not only on the organism that caused the infection but also on the location of the illness.

Certain cells, such as those found in the vaginal or upper respiratory tract, are easy prey for viruses. For example, the virus that causes rabies specifically attacks the nervous system. Warts are caused by some viruses that infect skin cells and cause growth.

Others attack a more diverse set of cells, resulting in many symptoms. A virus that causes influenza might result in symptoms such as a runny nose, aching muscles, and an upset stomach.

At the site of the infection, a person with a bacterial infection will frequently exhibit symptoms such as redness, heat, swelling, fever, and discomfort. Additionally, the infected person's lymph glands may swell.

A rash can sometimes identify a fungal infection of the skin. However, bacterial and viral infections can also bring skin problems and rashes.

Prion infections typically manifest themselves with a sudden onset of brain injury, memory loss, and cognitive impairments. They can also trigger the accumulation of plaque in the brain, which leads to the eating away of this organ.

Lists of Common Infections

A list of some of the most prevalent illnesses and infections that adults and children deal with nowadays is useful. Although the lists are incomplete, I think they assist in highlighting the very real health risks we constantly face. The following is a list of some of the most prevalent illnesses and infections found in children, teenagers, and elderly people:

Common Infections in Children and Young Adults

- Chicken Pox
- Croup
- Immune System Problems
- Ear Infections
- Head Lice
- MRSA
- Pneumonia
- Ringworm

- Respiratory Syncytial Virus (RSV)
- Salmonella
- Scabies
- Sexually Transmitted Diseases (STDs)
- Sore Throats
- West Nile Virus
- Update Cold and Flu
- Whooping Cough

Common Infections in Older Adults

Bacterial Pneumonia Herpes Zoster (also known as shingles)
26 Influenza Urinary tract infections (UTI)

Foods that need to be avoided: "Is this Gluten-Free?"

Becoming conscious of the foods you put into your body is the most important action you can take while transitioning to a diet that excludes gluten. In addition to adhering to the gluten-free diet, which I will discuss in greater depth in Part II, I also started seeking fresh foods grown locally and organically. This was done in conjunction with the plan. We were interested in purchasing foods that hadn't been in transit for several days to get to the store. We were aware that the degree to which the vegetables and fruit retained their freshness determined the degree to which they retained their potential health benefits. Food that has been processed extensively typically contains more harmful chemicals and fewer nutrients that produce energy. I concluded that it is difficult to determine what ingredients have been used in the manufacturing of the meal; this makes it more likely that the food is unhealthy.

Seasonal meals are typically the healthiest foods available. Boxed, tinned, and dehydrated foods with a long shelf life typically contain fewer nutrients than their fresh counterparts and are filled with chemicals, color, and preservatives. Boxed goods also have a longer shelf life.

Whole foods are the only source of the healthy proteins, carbs, and good fats that our body needs. While nutritional supplements can satisfy some of our dietary requirements, they cannot meet all of them. After several days of eating processed meals, I will feel exhausted and unmotivated due to the diet.

What is a Gluten-Free Diet?

A diet that does not include any foods that contain gluten is referred to as a gluten-free diet. The grains wheat, barley, rye, and triticale all contain a protein known as gluten (a cross between wheat and rye).

Celiac disease and other medical disorders related to gluten can only be managed effectively by consuming foods that do not contain gluten.

People not diagnosed with a medical problem related to gluten often follow a gluten-free diet because of its popularity. Although the diet is said to have benefits such as enhanced health, weight loss, and increased energy, additional research is required to verify these claims.

Gluten is the causative agent in the autoimmune illness known as celiac disease. This condition occurs when the immune system overreacts and causes damage to the lining of the small intestine. Because of this damage, over time, the body cannot absorb nutrients from the food it consumes. Celiac disease is an autoimmune condition and a type of inflammatory disease.

Even though there is no damage to the tissues of the small intestine, people with non-celiac gluten sensitivity still experience some of the signs and symptoms associated with celiac disease. These signs and symptoms include abdominal pain, bloating, diarrhea, constipation, "foggy brain," rash, and headaches.

Gluten ataxia is an autoimmune illness that causes muscle control and voluntary muscular movement problems. Certain nerve tissues are affected by gluten ataxia, which causes the disorder.

Wheat allergy is similar to other food allergies. It is caused by the immune system's mistaken identification of gluten or another protein contained in wheat as a pathogen, such as a virus or bacteria, that causes disease. The immune system produces an antibody in reaction to the protein, which triggers a response from the immune system, which may result in congestion, breathing difficulties, and other symptoms.

A healthy diet can include many of the following foods that are naturally free of gluten:

- Fruits and vegetables
- Raw nuts, seeds, beans, and other legumes.
- Eggs
- Lean cuts of meat, fish, and poultry that have not been overly processed

The Complete Anti-Inflammatory Diet for Beginners

The following grains, starches, and flours are examples of those that can be included in a gluten-free diet:

- Amaranth
- Arrowroot
- Buckwheat
- Corn — cornmeal, grits, and polenta labeled gluten-free
- Flax
- Gluten-free flours — rice, soy, corn, potato, and bean flours
- Hominy (corn)
- Millet
- Quinoa
- Rice, including wild rice
- Sorghum
- Soy
- Tapioca (cassava root)
- Teff

Steer clear of any foods and beverages that include the following ingredients:

- Wheat
- Barley
- Rye

- Triticale — a cross between wheat and rye
- Oats, in some cases

Even though oats do not contain gluten naturally, they could become contaminated with wheat, barley, or rye during manufacturing. Oats and oat-based goods marketed as gluten-free have not been subjected to cross-contamination. However, certain people suffer from celiac disease and cannot handle oats classified as gluten-free.

Chapter Five: Processed Foods and Its Dangers

There is evidence that consuming processed foods, such as ready-made meals, baked goods, and processed meats, may harm one's health.

A certain amount of processing is necessary for most foods, yet the body can still benefit from eating some processed meals.

However, meals that have been chemically processed, also known as ultra-processed foods, tend to contain a high amount of sugar, artificial chemicals, refined carbs, and trans fats. As a consequence of this, they are a significant factor in the growing rates of obesity and sickness all across the world.

Emma Collins

In the most recent decades, there has been a significant rise in the consumption of ultra-processed foods worldwide. In many parts of the world, consuming these foods currently makes up 25 and 60 percent of a person's daily energy intake.

What are Processed Foods?

Because most foods have been processed in some form, the term "processed food" might lead to some misunderstandings.

Foods do not inherently become less healthy just because they have been subjected to mechanical processing, such as grinding beef, boiling vegetables, or pasteurizing meals. If the preparation does not include any additional chemicals or substances, the food's health is not often compromised by the preparation.

However, there is a distinction between processing through mechanical means and processing through chemical means.

Foods that have undergone chemical processing typically only contain refined components and man-made compounds, which have little nutritional value. Chemical flavoring compounds, pigments, and sweeteners are frequently included in their formulations.

In contrast to whole foods, these foods that have undergone extremely high levels of processing are frequently referred to as "cosmetic" foods.

The following are some instances of foods that have been ultra-processed:

- Meals that are ready-made or frozen
- Products made in the oven, including pizza, cakes, and other baked items
- Bundled loaves of bread
- Cheese products that have been treated
- Cereals served for breakfast
- Snacks of chips and crackers
- Confectionery and frozen treats
- Reconstituted meats, such as sausages, nuggets, fish fingers, and processed ham
- Sodas and other sweetened drinks

Are foods that have been processed unhealthy to eat?

Foods that have undergone extreme processing typically have a pleasant flavor and are quite affordable.

On the other hand, they typically include components that, if ingested in excessive quantities, could have adverse health effects, such as added sugar, salt, and saturated fats. These foods are also lower in dietary fiber and nutrient content than their whole-food counterparts.

A study on Ultra-processed food intake and risk of cardiovascular disease: prospective cohort study involving more than 100,000 participants discovered that eating 10% more ultra-processed foods was connected with an increased risk of cardiovascular disease, coronary heart disease, and cerebrovascular diseases of more than 10%.

After considering the subjects' total fiber intake, saturated fat, sodium, and sugar, the researchers arrived at this verdict.

According to a study conducted by the Association between consumption of ultra-processed foods and all-cause mortality: SUN prospective cohort study that included over 20,000 participants, eating more than four servings of processed food daily was associated with an elevated risk of death from all causes. The risk of death from any cause increased by 18% with each additional dish that was consumed.

Eating a diet consisting of highly processed foods may cause one to gain excess weight.

In the following, we will examine seven potential reasons why consuming processed meals may pose a greater danger to one's health.

Added sugar

Added sugar and high fructose corn syrup are common components of processed foods. Added sugar is high in calories but lacks the vital elements found in natural sugar.

Consuming an excessive amount of added sugar consistently may cause compulsive overeating. In addition, it has been related to several health issues, including type 2 diabetes and inflammatory disorders, metabolic syndrome, and obesity.

The majority of the added sugar that people consume comes from foods and beverages that have been processed. People typically consume far more sugar than they realize they are getting from soft drinks, making sweetened beverages a particularly significant source of the substance.

A simple and efficient strategy for making dietary changes that contribute to improved health is to reduce the amount of added sugar consumed. One example of this strategy would be to replace soda with carbonated water.

Emma Collins

Artificial Ingredients

On the back of the box for processed foods, you'll frequently find a list of ingredients that contains a lot of obscure ingredients. Some of them are man-made compounds that the producer has added to the food to make it taste better.

The following categories of chemicals can frequently be found in highly processed foods:

Additives that prevent the food from deteriorating too soon, such as preservatives, artificial coloring, chemical flavoring, and texturing ingredients. In addition, the labels on processed foods may not disclose the presence of dozens of other chemicals that may be present in the product.

One example of a proprietary mixture is something called "artificial flavor." The manufacturers are not required to reveal exactly what it means; in most cases, it refers to a combination of different compounds.

Even though the vast majority of food additives have passed safety tests conducted by official bodies, the usage of many of these compounds is still debated by medical professionals and academics.

Refined carbohydrates

Carbohydrates are an important factor in the overall composition of any diet. However, carbohydrates from whole foods have significantly more positive effects on one's health than processed carbohydrates.

Refined carbohydrates, also known as simple carbs, are broken down rapidly in the body, resulting in rapid increases in blood sugar and insulin levels. The subsequent dip in these levels can cause an individual to feel lethargic and hungry at the same time.

Consumption of refined carbohydrates is associated with an elevated risk due to the rapid rises and falls in blood sugar that these carbohydrates induce.

Foods that have undergone extensive processing are typically high in refined carbs.

These are some examples of healthy sources of carbohydrates:

- Whole grains
- Fruits
- Vegetables

Emma Collins

Low in Nutrients

Compared to whole meals or foods with only a small amount of processing, ultra-processed foods have an extremely low level of vital elements.

Sometimes, to make up for the nutrients lost during the manufacturing process, manufacturers will mix synthetic vitamins and mineral supplements. Whole foods, on the other hand, include extra chemicals that benefit health, but ultra-processed meals do not.

For instance, fruits, vegetables, and grains have beneficial plant components, such as those with antioxidant, anti-inflammatory, and anticarcinogenic properties. These compounds include carotenoids, flavonoids, anthocyanins, and tannins.

Eating whole foods, either unprocessed or just minimally processed, is the greatest method to ensure that you get all the key nutrients your body needs.

The Complete Anti-Inflammatory Diet for Beginners

A diet low in fiber

The benefits of dietary fiber to one's health are extensive and varied.

The digestion of carbs is slowed by the fiber, making people feel fuller on a diet that contains fewer calories. In addition to these benefits, it also performs the prebiotic function, meaning that it provides food for the beneficial bacteria found in the digestive tract and can assist in improving cardiovascular health.

Most ultra-processed foods contain relatively little fiber due to natural fiber removal.

Foods high in fiber that are healthy include:

- Legumes
- Fruits
- Vegetables
- Nuts
- Seeds

Quick calories

The processing done to meals by their makers makes them relatively simple to chew and swallow.

Ultra-processed foods require less energy to eat and digest than whole meals or foods with a lower processing level because a significant portion of the fiber is removed during the processing step.

Because of this, consuming a greater quantity of these goods in a shorter amount of time is much simpler. When a person does this, rather than eating whole foods as they normally would, they take in more calories yet expend a lower amount of energy in the digestive process.

Because of this, a person's likelihood of taking in more calories than they burn increases, resulting in accidental weight gain.

Trans fats

Foods that have undergone extreme processing are frequently heavy in unhealthy and inexpensive fats. For instance, they frequently contain refined seed or vegetable oils, are typically simple to apply, relatively inexpensive, and can keep for a considerable amount of time.

Manufacturers produce artificial trans fats by adding hydrogen to liquid vegetable oils, which causes the oils to become more solid.

Trans fats exacerbate the inflammation that occurs throughout the body. In addition, they cause an increase in low-density lipoprotein, commonly known as "bad" cholesterol, while causing a decrease in high-density lipoprotein, generally known as "good" cholesterol.

Consuming foods containing trans fats is linked to an increased likelihood of developing cardiovascular disease, stroke, and type 2 diabetes. For instance, a study published in 2019 found that a 2% increase in the proportion of one's total caloric intake that comes from trans fats is associated with a 23% increase in one's risk of developing cardiovascular disease.

Avoiding processed foods is the most effective strategy for staying away from refined oils and trans fats. People can substitute these for other foods that are better for their health, such as olive oil or coconut oil.

Emma Collins

Sugar and Inflammation

People who consume a lot of refined sugar may be putting themselves at a greater risk of developing a chronic inflammatory condition. According to research, inflammatory indicators in people's blood diminish when they consume less sugar in their diet and beverages.

A diet heavy in sugar can have adverse consequences on health, including raising the chance of developing chronic diseases, contributing to weight gain, and accelerating tooth decay. It is also possible for this to develop in chronic inflammation, a condition in which the immune system of the body becomes activated, causing damage to healthy cells.

The link between sugar and inflammation

Inflammation may be affected by consuming a diet that is high in sugar.

According to research about the effects of diet on inflammation: emphasis on metabolic syndrome, one's choice of diet can substantially influence the level of inflammation within the body. While certain foods might make inflammation worse, others can make it better. A diet heavy in sugar may be one of the primary factors contributing to ongoing inflammation.

The Complete Anti-Inflammatory Diet for Beginners

According to a recent meta-analysis (2018) on the Effect of Dietary Sugar Intake on Biomarkers of Subclinical Inflammation: A Systematic Review and Meta-Analysis of Intervention Studies, considerable research has found a connection between ingesting a greater quantity of dietary sugar, particularly sugary drinks, and chronic inflammation. Those whose diets contain more sugar have a higher concentration of inflammatory indicators in their blood, including a marker known as C-reactive protein.

A 2014 study on Decreased consumption of sugar-sweetened beverages improved selected biomarkers of chronic disease risk among US adults: 1999 to 2010 found out those who lowered the amount of sugar-sweetened beverages had lower levels of inflammatory markers in their blood. These findings provide evidence in support of the hypothesis that eating sugar can bring about inflammation.

Researchers have endeavored to understand the mechanism by which sugar brings about inflammation. The liver's generation of free fatty acids is prompted by sugar consumption. When the body digests these free fatty acids, the leftover substances can potentially start inflammatory processes.

Different types of sugar may be responsible for varying degrees of inflammation. For example, a few pieces of study have suggested that fructose might be more likely to promote inflammation than glucose. However, since a systematic review discovered that there is no difference in inflammation caused by fructose and glucose, there is a need for additional research.

In addition, the researchers did not find any changes in the levels of inflammatory variables between the groups that consumed high fructose corn syrup and those that consumed sucrose. Because of the low quality of the studies and the relatively small sample sizes, it is important to do additional research to verify these findings.

Other ways Sugar can Affect the Body.

Consuming sugar over a prolonged period has a variety of adverse impacts on the body, including an increased chance of chronic inflammation, obesity, diabetes, and tooth decay.

Sucrose and fructose can cause plaque on a person's teeth, leading to tooth decay and cavities. Sugar is food for the cavity-causing bacteria in your mouth. Sugary foods encourage the growth of germs in the mouth, which in turn wears down tooth enamel and can lead to cavities.

Sugar-sweetened beverages can add many calories to one's diet; nevertheless, doing so does not help a person feel fuller. This temporary increase in calorie consumption may ultimately result in long-term weight gain. Instead, the calories that come from solid foods cause people to feel fuller and help them eat less.

Emma Collins

Part II: The Heart of the Matter – Gluten-Free Living

Emma Collins

The Complete Anti-Inflammatory Diet for Beginners

Introduction

If you're one of the estimated 3 million Americans with celiac disease, you know that going gluten-free is essential to your health. But even if you don't have celiac disease, you may benefit from giving up gluten.

There's growing evidence that gluten can cause inflammation in the body, and that's a problem even if you don't have celiac disease. Inflammation has been linked to various health problems, including heart disease, arthritis, and depression.

So, if you're considering going gluten-free, it's worth considering whether it could help improve your overall health. Here's what you need to know about the link between gluten and inflammation.

Emma Collins

Chapter Six: Nutritional Necessities

The Importance of a Balanced Diet in Many Inflammatory Conditions

Before we go any further, let's briefly go through the basic factors contributing to inflammation to appreciate the value of maintaining a healthy diet. Infection, allergies, environmental toxins, physical damage, emotional trauma, dietary deficiencies, and excesses are some of the most prevalent causes of inflammation. As we have already mentioned, some of the most common types of inflammation include:

Infection: A fungus, bacteria, yeast, virus, or other parasites will attack the system in the event of an infection. Infections can develop in the system.

The Complete Anti-Inflammatory Diet for Beginners

The inflammation that results from the immune system's response to an infection serves as a preparation for war against the pathogen.

An allergic reaction takes place, as was mentioned before, when the body's immune system overreacts to any chemical, whether it is hazardous or not, that has the potential to be harmful to the body. This can include both harmful and innocuous substances. This could be caused by anything, from a certain dish to an insect bite. Inflammation is the body's natural response to any threat and serves as a defense mechanism. There is a spectrum of possible reactions, from moderate to severe.

Injury and Toxicity: Cells subjected to either chemical or physical irritants are more likely to experience inflammation. There are several toxins (pesticides, tobacco, medicines, asbestos, and so on) that have the potential to cause damage to the tissues of the body. Continuous exposure often results in inflammation as a strategy to protect and mend injured areas. This is done to protect the body from further damage. The body's natural response to damaged cells and tissues, inflammation aids in the body's ability to mend and restore these areas.

Emotional Abuse Both stress and worry have the potential to hurt the body. Their mental state can directly impact the physical state of a person. When a person is subjected to emotional stress, their body releases increased quantities of cortisone hormones and adrenaline, which leads to an imbalance and inflammation. Growing older tends to make the problem much more severe. The body is frequently unprepared to deal with the onslaught that it is experiencing. When a person is healthy, their body can better eliminate toxins through processes such as flushing and sweating.

Insufficiency in Nutrition and Overconsumption of Nutrition: Nutritional inconsistencies are frequently linked to hormonal abnormalities, a strained immune system, and inflammation in the body. Suppose you don't get enough of certain nutrients, such as the right kinds of protein, lipids, carbohydrates, vitamins, and minerals. In that case, it's possible that your body won't have enough of the nutrients it needs to repair damaged cells and tissues.

On the other hand, consuming an excessive amount of particular foods might result in a nutritional imbalance, which can stress the tissues and organs of the body. As can be seen, several elements are at play, including mental health, physical activity, environmental circumstances, lifestyle factors, genetic predisposition, and food. When we make it a priority to lessen the number of toxins our family is exposed to, we not only become more conscientious of how we treat our bodies and pay closer attention to what we eat, but we also give ourselves a greater capacity to deal with potentially dangerous circumstances. In the second part of this book, "Part II," we will discuss the significance of reducing inflammation through gaining an awareness of our bodies nutritional requirements and the gluten-free diet.

Difference between True Hunger and Cravings

Hunger is a built-in device that alerts us to our bodies' specific nutritional requirements at any given time. A person may suffer from a nutritional deficiency if they have food cravings. For instance, a need for salty foods may indicate a salt deficit in the body. However, many food cravings are caused by an emotional component. It is common for people to develop cravings for a certain type of food when they are dieting and trying to eliminate that food from their diet. Take, for instance, the fact that you have been munching on a bag of chips while working on your computer in the evening. If you decide to eliminate that activity from your daily routine, you should be prepared for a time during which you will have an intense desire for chips. If the thought of eating an apple satisfies the urge, then it is probable that what you are going through is a real hunger and not just a need for chips.

This is a helpful technique to identify whether or not you are going through real hunger instead of a craving for chips. If nothing else will satisfy you, you almost certainly have an appetite for some kind of food. (A medical evaluation can sometimes be necessary because of an underlying condition.) When people eat for the right reasons, they often only consume food when they are, starving, and they stop eating when they are satiated rather than when they have reached an uncomfortable level of fullness. A diet that is generally gratifying will include nutritious foods, yet at the same time, it will not exclude particularly pleasurable items.

On the other hand, when a person allows themselves to be controlled by their cravings for food, they have a greater propensity to put on weight, overeat, and experience a decline in their nutritional status. A chart that differentiates between the indicators of actual hunger and cravings and the signs of emotional food cravings may be found below. Bear in mind that different people react differently to hunger in different ways.

Know How to Keep Track of your Food Intake

The simplest way to stay in tune with your body is by keeping a food journal. A food journal allows you to keep track of your eating habits. You can record how you feel before, during, and after eating. Keep track of how hungry you are at various stages throughout the day. By getting in touch with triggers and patterns, you'll soon be able to recognize and avoid giving in to emotional cravings. If emotions get the best of you, you may be able to replace that bag of chips with sensible, gluten-free snacks. Emotions and eating patterns are closely linked. Your journal will help to make connections between emotions and eating habits. With practice, you can replace eating foods that cause inflammation with gluten-free foods that help to promote better health. Gluten-free recipes and meal plans included in this book will provide healthy alternatives. As you tune into your true nutritional needs, you are likely to feel healthier in every way.

Why Anti-Inflammatory Diets?

As we can see, our eating habits involve a complicated web of many elements. Our entire system influences how we feel about food and the meal itself. The nutrients we take in affect all the organs in our body and significantly affect our immune system. The immune system is composed of an intricate network of different components. Each of the components must receive the necessary maintenance. If they are not, the process as a whole may be thrown off-kilter. When our immune systems aren't functioning properly, we make ourselves considerably more vulnerable to various illnesses and other health issues. If you have a weak immune system, you will be less able to fend off the attack of a wide variety of pathogens that are harmful to you. Chronic inflammation, illness, and other autoimmune reactions are all potential outcomes of such an imbalance, which allows for the unrestrained invasion of undesirable organisms. A diet that reduces inflammation helps prevent such an imbalance and prepares the body for healing and achieving optimal health. Both academic study and personal experiences have shown that following a diet that reduces inflammation confers several health benefits to the body.

A significant benefit of following an anti-inflammatory diet is that it makes it easier to steer clear of foods that are known to provoke allergic reactions within the body. In addition, it stops many unwelcome substances from entering our systems. A strong immune system can protect the body against the negative effects of toxins, hormones, and antibiotic residues. A diet that reduces inflammation is good because it emphasizes consuming unprocessed, natural foods. Foods that have undergone excessive processing are either avoided or limited. At the same time, foods that are good for us and are high in beneficial nutrients are being introduced into our system. Digestion is made easier, and less damage is done to the body while following a diet that reduces inflammation. When the circulatory and digestive systems are supplied with the appropriate proportion of nutrients, they are not required to break down foods that are tough to digest. It is then able to metabolize the meals that are necessary for maintaining optimum health. Nutrients do not have to process in difficult-to-digest foods. It is freed up to metabolize foods that ensure optimal health.

Can a Diet Affect Inflammation?

After performing a ton of research on the subject, I am convinced that one's diet can influence inflammation. In this book, I provide a diet program that combines many aspects of an anti-inflammatory diet with a gluten-free diet. This diet program is intended to help people who suffer from inflammatory conditions. A quick reminder that different people have different reactions to the same foods. Incorporating any number of these dietary tenets into one's lifestyle can, in my opinion, contribute to positive and long-term improvements in one's health. As we will see, removing gluten from one's diet, particularly highly processed white flour and sugar, will instantly enhance one's overall health.

In addition, removing highly processed meats from the diet (many of which contain gluten as an additive) enables the system to function without hiccups. Immediate improvements in my family's overall health were observed after we made some lifestyle changes. On the other hand, the effects can show up in a more piecemeal fashion for certain people. If you have a chronic ailment and have seen a doctor about it, switching to a gluten-free and anti-inflammatory diet may be the first step toward better health. A diet that helps reduce inflammation can offer many health benefits. This book recommends cutting out foods that might contribute to your health problems and then slowly returning them to your diet. I hope that you will experience many of the same benefits to your health that I have by keeping a daily food log and adhering to these habits. In the following chapters, we will go into further detail on various useful anti-inflammatory and gluten-free ideas that you can easily include in your daily diet and wellness regimen.

When you go to the grocery store, your decisions can affect the inflammation throughout your body. However, there are several things that researchers have figured out about how food might influence the inflammatory processes that occur inside the body.

According to research, the food you consume can affect the levels of C-reactive protein (CRP), a marker for inflammation, found in your blood. This may be because certain meals, like processed sweets, release inflammatory messengers, increasing the risk of chronic inflammation. Your body can better combat oxidative stress, which is a potential driver of inflammation when you eat other nutrients like fruits and vegetables.

The good news is that meals that assist reduce inflammation tend to be the same nutrients that help maintain your health in other areas. Therefore, paying attention to your diet to reduce inflammation does not have to be difficult or restrictive.

When to Expect Results

No miracle cure can be achieved by simply beginning an anti-inflammatory diet. The intensity of your intolerance and inflammation will determine the range of possible outcomes for you.

Give yourself three to six months to make changes to your diet and to begin to see results, just like me; "Drastic changes never lead to long-term success. You can start by making a few simple adjustments you are confident will significantly impact, and then gradually add more."

If you have a major reaction to a particular meal, you may see results in as little as two to three weeks after removing that food from your diet. This is only the case if you eliminate the food.

I believe that this can be a highly encouraging and inspiring factor for people.

Emma Collins

Simple guidelines to follow to reduce inflammation through diet

Eat more plants. Whole plant foods include the nutrient anti-inflammatory agents necessary for your body. Therefore, the best way to begin is by consuming various fruits, vegetables, whole grains, and legumes in a rainbow of colors.

Pay attention to antioxidants. They can prevent, postpone, or heal some types of damage that can occur to cells and tissues. They can be found in various brightly colored fruits and vegetables, such as berries, leafy greens, beets, avocados, beans, and lentils. Whole grains, turmeric, ginger, and green tea.

Get your Omega-3s. The inflammatory process in your body is partially controlled by omega-3 fatty acids, which also have the potential to help regulate the discomfort that is associated with inflammation. You can get these good fats from fish like salmon, tuna, and mackerel, as well as in smaller amounts from walnuts, pecans, ground flaxseed, and soy. Salmon and mackerel are all examples of seafood.

Reduce your intake of red meat. The consumption of red meat may contribute to inflammation. Do you enjoy eating hamburgers? Set your sights on an attainable objective. You may try having fish, almonds, or a protein-based dish made from soy a few times per week instead of beef for lunch.

Reduce your consumption of processed foods. Offenders contributing to inflammation include sugary cereals and drinks, deep-fried foods, and baked goods. They may contain a significant amount of harmful fats, which have been related to inflammatory responses. Eating whole fruits, vegetables, grains, and beans might be a time-efficient option if you plan and prepare food for numerous meals.

Anti-Inflammatory Diet Principles

Our decisions now affect our health, potentially affecting us in the coming years. As our children become older, various changes occur within their bodies simultaneously. Even young adults' brains, immune systems, and sensitive nerve systems are still maturing and developing. The greatest way to increase this process is through consuming nutritious foods and adopting healthy behaviors. The anti-inflammatory and gluten-free diets are founded on the same foundation, which encourages limiting exposure to potentially harmful chemicals and centering one's daily diet around consuming nutritious foods. If we start teaching the fundamentals of a healthy lifestyle from a younger age, we will have a better chance of avoiding chronic diseases in the future and leading fuller, more vibrant lives. In addition to concentrating on leading a healthy life, I firmly believe we should work to improve our children's emotional well-being. Through our deeds and our words, we demonstrate to our children our love for them and our faith in their potential as individuals. I feel it's important to point out that even very minor diseases in youngsters can sometimes assist the body's immune system to get stronger. The capacity of our children to avoid getting sick naturally improves as they grow older. Their immune system is "training" and maturing at the same time. If we try to suppress the immune system by using needless suppressants, we will affect the body's natural ability to defend itself against potential dangers. We should work toward establishing a natural equilibrium, which can be facilitated by consuming a healthy and beneficial diet for the body's immune system.

Chapter Seven: The Anti-Inflammation Diet

Lifestyle Alert: Gluten-Free Protein

Living gluten-free changes almost every aspect of our life. We needed to rethink the foods we were eating and how we shopped, selected recipes, and prepared our family's meals. In the next few chapters, I have provided a four-week meal plan, shopping guides, and recipes that will help you along your path to living a gluten-free and anti-inflammatory diet. If you are one of the countless people who suffer from digestive difficulties, chronic disease, allergies, sleeping problems, skin problems, and mood swings, this "Lifestyle Alert: Gluten Free" diet may be exactly what you are looking for.

Emma Collins

Types of Fats

One nutrient that can be found in food is called dietary fat. The word "fat" used to be considered offensive when discussing nutrition. Many years ago, your physician probably advised you to reduce or eliminate the amount of fat in your diet to avoid gaining weight and developing serious health complications like heart disease and diabetes. These days, medical professionals are aware that not all fats are harmful. Your cholesterol level can be lowered by eating certain fats, contributing to your overall health. You need some fat in your diet.

Your body relies on fats for a variety of critical processes, and their advantages include:

- Give you energy
- Maintain a warm body temperature.
- Develop your cells and guard your organs.
- Improve your body's ability to absorb nutrients from the diet.
- Produce hormones that will assist your body in functioning appropriately.

The goal is to ensure that your diet contains a healthy balance of fats and other nutrients. Consume the types and amounts of fats that are the healthiest for you. The most beneficial fats are those that are unsaturated. Saturated and trans fats are generally less healthy than their unsaturated counterparts.

Saturated and Unsaturated Fats

The chemical structure of various dietary lipids differentiates them from one another. All fats share the same structure, consisting of a series of carbon atoms bound to hydrogen atoms and linked together in a chain.

Saturated fats have carbon atoms that are completely coated, or "saturated," with hydrogen atoms. This gives saturated fats their name. Because of this, they are now solid when they are at room temperature.

Fewer hydrogen atoms are covalently bonded to carbon atoms in unsaturated lipids than in saturated fats. These lipids are liquid even when the temperature is room temperature.

Emma Collins

Saturated fats

A diet that is high in saturated fats can cause your total cholesterol to rise and can shift the balance of cholesterol in your body toward the more dangerous LDL cholesterol. This can cause blockages in the arteries of your heart and other parts of your body. Your chance of developing heart disease increases with high LDL cholesterol.

The following are examples of foods that contain saturated fat:

- Red meat like beef, lamb, and pork
- Chicken and other types of poultry with their skins intact
- Dairy items are made from whole milk, such as milk, cheese, and ice cream.
- Butter
- Eggs
- Coconut and palm

Concerning saturated fats, there is some disagreement amongst medical professionals. According to the findings of several studies, there is no evidence that these fats contribute directly to the development of heart disease. And it's possible that certain kinds of saturated fat, like the one found in milk, are healthier for you than others, like the kind found in red meat.

The American Heart Association suggests consuming no more than 5% or 6% of your total daily calories from saturated fat. You should consume less than 10% of your calories from saturated fat. If you consume 2,000 calories daily, the maximum amount of saturated fat you should consume is equivalent to 120 or 13 grams.

Considering what you consume in place of saturated fat in your diet is important. For instance, consuming polyunsaturated rather than saturated fats may reduce the risk of cardiovascular disease. However, replacing saturated fats with carbs may increase the risk of developing cardiovascular disease.

Unsaturated fats

Vegetables, nuts, and seafood are the diet's primary sources of unsaturated fats. They are in a liquid state when the room temperature is reached. Medical professionals recommend consuming these fats instead of saturated and trans fats. This is because these fats are healthy for your heart and the rest of your body.

There are two varieties of unsaturated fats:

Emma Collins

One of the chemical bonds of monounsaturated fatty acids is unsaturated. When placed in the refrigerator, oils containing these fats transform into a solid state, despite being liquid at room temperature.

Foods such as those listed below are good sources of monounsaturated fats.

- Avocados
- oils derived from olives, canola, and peanuts
- Nuts of several kinds, including almonds, hazelnuts, pecans, and others.

Polyunsaturated fats are characterized by the presence of several unsaturated chemical linkages. Polyunsaturated oils do not solidify under any temperature, including room temperature and the refrigerator.

Foods such as those listed below are good sources of polyunsaturated fat.

- Oils extracted from flaxseed, corn, soybeans, and sunflowers
- Walnuts
- Flaxseeds
- Fatty fish such as salmon, tuna, and others

The Complete Anti-Inflammatory Diet for Beginners

Omega-3 fatty acids and omega-6 fatty acids are the two varieties of polyunsaturated fats.

There are three different types of omega-3 fatty acids:

Eicosapentaenoic acid (EPA) is primarily found in fish.
Docosahexaenoic acid (DHA) is also primarily found in fish.
Alpha-linolenic acid (ALA) is primarily found in plant sources such as flaxseed, vegetable oils, and nuts.

According to several studies, eating fish rich in omega-3 fatty acids can lower your risk of cardiovascular disease. Taking omega-3 pills, on the other hand, could not have the same beneficial effect. In addition, scientists are investigating whether or not omega-3 fatty acids can help prevent or halt the progression of Alzheimer's disease and other forms of dementia.

Because your body cannot produce these critical fats on its own, you must obtain them through your diet. At least twice a week, you should eat fatty fish such as salmon, mackerel, and herring to ensure that your diet contains an adequate amount of omega-3 fatty acids.

Foods such as dark leafy green vegetables, seeds, nuts, and vegetable oils are all good sources of omega-6 fatty acids. Omega-6 fatty acids were once thought to be a contributing factor in the development of heart disease by medical professionals. There is evidence to show that these fatty acids are beneficial to one's heart.

The American Heart Association recommends that you acquire between 5 and 10 percent of your daily calorie intake from omega-6 fatty acids. The diets of the majority of people already provide them with this quantity.

Trans Fats

In foods derived from animals, such as meat and milk, naturally occurring quantities of trans fats can be found. However, the majority of trans fats are produced by an industrial method. Food manufacturers add hydrogen to the oils to make liquid vegetable oils solid at room temperature. This helps foods maintain their freshness for longer. In addition to that, it improves both the taste and the texture of the food.

There is a possibility that the following foods contain trans fats:

- Fried dishes like French fries and other favorites
- Other baked foods besides cakes, pies, biscuits, cookies, crackers, and doughnuts.
- Margarine available in sticks or tubs

- Popcorn made in a microwave
- Frozen pizza

Although trans fats may have a pleasant flavor, it is not healthy to consume them. Your risk of developing cardiovascular disease, stroke, and type 2 diabetes increases when you consume this sort of bad fat, which also elevates your LDL cholesterol level. It does this by bringing down your "good" HDL cholesterol. Trans fats should account for no more than one percent of your daily caloric intake, as per the recommendation of the American Heart Association. Several areas have completely outlawed trans fats.

Are foods without trans fats healthier than other foods?

Not necessarily. Even though they do not contain trans fats, some foods may contain dangerous saturated fat. They could have a high concentration of sugar and salt, both of which are detrimental to your health. Before consuming any packaged or processed goods, thoroughly read the labels.

The main line is that you should receive most of your fats from unsaturated sources if you want to keep your heart and the rest of you healthy. And ensure that most of your daily calories come from nutritious meals low in fat, such as vegetables, fruits, and whole grains, as well as lean proteins like fish and chicken without the skin.

Omega-6 Importance

Fatty acids with the omega-6 designation are considered essential fatty acids. They are essential for human health, but the body cannot produce them independently. You can only get them through the consumption of food. In addition to omega-3 fatty acids, omega-6 fatty acids are extremely important to the proper functioning of the brain and proper growth and development. Omega-6s are a form of polyunsaturated fatty acid (PUFA). Its benefits include promoting healthy skin and hair growth, maintaining strong bones, controlling metabolism, and keeping the reproductive system in good working order.

Fatty acids omega-3 and omega-6 should be present in about equal amounts in a diet that is considered healthy. Inflammation can be mitigated, in part, by omega-3 fatty acids, whereas some omega-6 fatty acids tend to exacerbate the condition. There is evidence from a few research that suggests increased consumption of omega-6 fatty acids may be associated with complicated regional pain syndrome. The average diet in the United States often ranges from 14 to 25 times the amount of omega-6 fatty acids as omega-3 fatty acids.

On the other hand, the Mediterranean diet features a more favorable proportion of omega-3 to omega-6 fatty acids in its overall composition. Studies have shown that persons who eat like that in the Mediterranean have a lower risk of developing heart disease. The Mediterranean diet does not include a significant amount of meat (which is high in omega-6 fatty acids, although grass-fed beef has a more favorable omega-3 to omega-6 fatty acid ratio), and it emphasizes foods that are rich in omega-3 fatty acids. These foods include whole grains, fresh fruits and vegetables, fish, olive oil, garlic, and moderate consumption of wine.

There are several distinct kinds of omega-6 fatty acids, and not all of them are associated with increased inflammation. It is important not to confuse linoleic acid (LA), a type of omega-6 fatty acid, with alpha-linolenic acid (ALA), a type of omega-3 fatty acid. The majority of omega-6 fatty acids in the diet originate from vegetable oils. Within the body, linoleic acid is changed into gamma-linolenic acid, also known as GLA. After that, it can further decompose into arachidonic acid (AA). Evening primrose oil (often referred to as EPO), borage oil, and black currant seed oil are just a few plant-based oils containing GLA.

It's possible that GLA can help reduce inflammation. A significant portion of the GLA that is consumed in the form of a supplement is transformed into an anti-inflammatory compound called DGLA. GLA can be converted into DGLA more effectively if sufficient amounts of certain minerals are present in the body. These nutrients include magnesium, zinc, and vitamins C, B3, and B6.

Uses

The following are some health problems in which omega-6 fatty acids might be beneficial:

Neuropathy caused by diabetes

Some research suggests that persons with diabetic neuropathy who take gamma-linolenic acid (GLA) for at least six months may reduce nerve pain symptoms. People with a good handle on their blood sugar may find that GLA is more beneficial than others who have a poor handle on their blood sugar.

Arthritis rheumatoid of the knee (RA)

The Complete Anti-Inflammatory Diet for Beginners

The results of studies on whether evening primrose oil (EPO) helps alleviate symptoms of rheumatoid arthritis are varied. However, other studies have shown that EPO did not affect pain, edema, or morning stiffness. The preliminary evidence suggests that EPO may lessen these symptoms. Treating arthritis symptoms with GLA could take anywhere from one to three months for the benefits to become apparent. It is improbable that EPO would be effective in halting the progression of the disease. So joint injury would still occur.

Allergies

Omega-6 fatty acids found in food or supplements, such as GLA derived from EPO or other sources, have a long tradition of using alternative medicine to treat allergic reactions. It seems that the levels of GLA in breast milk and blood are lower in women predisposed to allergic reactions. However, there is insufficient evidence from scientific studies to suggest that consuming GLA can help alleviate the symptoms of allergies. We require research investigations that have been carefully carried out.

Consult your physician before attempting to use GLA as a treatment for your allergies so that you can assess if it is safe for you to do so. The next step is to carefully monitor your symptoms of allergies to look for any evidence of improvement.

ADHD

According to several clinical investigations, children with ADHD have lower amounts of EFAs overall, including omega-6s and omega-3s. The proper operation of the brain and behavior depends on the presence of EFAs. Despite methodological flaws, several studies have found that ingesting fish oil, which is rich in omega-3 fatty acids, can help lessen the symptoms of attention deficit hyperactivity disorder (ADHD). Most research on EPO concluded that it was no more effective than a placebo at reducing symptoms.

Cancer of the breast

Tamoxifen is a medicine that is used to treat estrogen-sensitive breast cancer. One study indicated that women with breast cancer who took GLA had a greater response to tamoxifen (than those who took only tamoxifen). According to the findings of other studies, GLA reduces the amount of tumor activity in breast cancer cell lines. There is some evidence from research to suggest that eating a diet high in omega-6 fatty acids may increase the risk of developing breast cancer. DO NOT add fatty acid supplements, or any other supplements, to your treatment program for breast cancer unless your physician specifically permits you.

Eczema

There is a lack of consensus on whether or not EPO can assist in alleviating the symptoms of eczema. There was some evidence of benefit from preliminary research, but the studies were not adequately constructed. In further investigations, researchers looked at participants who took EPO for 16 to 24 weeks and found that their symptoms did not improve. If you are interested in trying EPO, you should consult your physician to find out whether or not it is safe for you to do so.

Hypertension

There is some evidence to suggest that gamma-linolenic acid (GLA) may help lower high blood pressure, either on its own or in conjunction with omega-3 fatty acids found in fish oil, specifically eicosapentaenoic acid (EPA) and docosahexaenoic acid (DHA). This may be the case whether GLA is taken alone or in combination with these acids (DHA). One study found that men with borderline high blood pressure who took 6 grams of blackcurrant oil had a lower diastolic blood pressure than those who received a placebo. This drop was seen in the men's diastolic blood pressure.

In another study, participants with intermittent claudication, which manifests as pain in the legs when walking and is brought on by obstructions in the blood arteries, were investigated. Those who took GLA and EPA together had lower systolic blood pressure than those who received a placebo, indicating that the combination reduced blood pressure.

Menopausal symptoms

EPO has recently seen a surge in popularity as a treatment for the hot flashes common during menopause. But the research that has been done so far has not concluded. If you wish to try EPO to treat your hot flashes and night sweats, you should first consult your physician to ensure that it is safe and appropriate for you.

Ache in the breasts (mastalgia)

In individuals who suffer from cyclic mastalgia, there is evidence to suggest that EPO may lessen the severity of breast pain and tenderness. People who suffer from noncyclic mastalgia may also find that it helps somewhat alleviate their symptoms. On the other hand, it does not appear to be helpful for moderate to severe breast pain.

Multiple sclerosis (MS)

Although there is no scientific evidence that it is effective, EPO has been suggested as a supplementary treatment (in addition to the usual medication) for multiple sclerosis (MS). MS patients interested in incorporating EPO into their existing treatment plans should consult with a qualified medical professional.

Osteoporosis

According to certain research findings, people who do not acquire enough essential fatty acids (especially EPA and GLA) are more prone to experience bone loss than individuals whose levels of these fatty acids are within the normal range. In a study including osteoporosis in women over 65, those who took EPA and GLA supplements showed a slower rate of bone loss over three years compared to those who took a placebo. A significant number of these ladies also improved their bone density.

Premenstrual syndrome (PMS)

Although most research has concluded that GLA has no effect, some women have reported that it has helped relieve the symptoms of PMS. Breast tenderness, feelings of depression, irritability, swelling, and bloating due to fluid retention are the symptoms that appear to improve the most.

Other symptoms that seem to improve include irritability and swelling from fluid retention.

Sources from the Diet

It is important to strike a healthy equilibrium between omega-6 and omega-3 fatty acids for one's overall well-being. The ratio of omega-6 to omega-3 fatty acids should fall somewhere in the range of 2:1 to 4:1; however, there are health educators who argue for even lower ratios. Oils derived from sunflower, safflower, soybeans, sesame, and corn are all good sources of omega-6 fatty acids. Supplements are typically unnecessary because the typical diet already contains enough omega-6 fatty acids. People who suffer from certain illnesses, including eczema, psoriasis, arthritis, diabetes, or breast pain (mastalgia), may wish to discuss the possibility of taking omega-6 supplements with their primary care physicians.

How you Can Prevent Omega-6 Fats from Promoting Inflammation (Tips)

Most diets include an excessive omega-6 but only a small amount of omega-3 fats. According to the findings of recent studies, an omega-6 to omega-3 fat ratio of approximately 2:1 may be able to reduce levels of inflammation significantly. In addition, studies have shown that the levels of inflammation in people whose diets contain a greater ratio of omega-3 fats to other types of fats are lower. Most foods that contain grains, baked goods, confectionery, and snack foods also contain omega-6 fats. Where exactly do all of these omega-6 fats originate?

Most of the omega-6 fats that people consume are derived from sweets, baked products, cereals, and snack foods. It is estimated that as much as 20% of the daily calorie consumption of the typical American comes from soybean oil, a substance that is included in most processed goods. Omega-6 consumption can also be reduced by reading food labels and consuming fewer foods. Simply lowering our intake of omega-6 fats helps us strengthen our immune systems by causing an increase in the creation of cells that fight inflammation throughout the body. Checking the labels is imperative at this point. Eat fewer meals high in omega-6 fats and focus on getting more omega-3 fats instead. This will help you feel more energized. Vegetables and fruits that are good for you, together with goods that do not contain gluten, can boost your stamina while protecting you against inflammation, which can cause allergic reactions, illness, and disease.

Note: You should note that the consumption of omega-6 fats is not entirely bad. However, consuming too many omega-6 fats more than omega-3 fats is bad for your health. The suggested ratio is ratio 2:1. You should consume twice as much omega 3 fats as you consume omega 6 fats. The recommended daily intake of omega-6 fats According to the Food and Nutrition Board of the U.S. Institute of Medicine, the adequate intake of omega-6s per day is 17 grams for males and 12 grams for females ages 19–50 years.

Lists of Foods that Help Decrease Inflammation

My overarching goal is to facilitate a healthy lifestyle for you to lead. We have discussed the potential repercussions of inflammation and gained some knowledge about good proteins and lipids. The following lists various so-called "superfoods" developed to combat inflammation.

The Complete Anti-Inflammatory Diet for Beginners

Almonds - Almonds are a source of protein, fiber, healthy fats, and antioxidants, in addition to a meal containing fiber. (Daily, eating one to two handfuls of almonds free of salt, gluten, and sugar is associated with numerous health advantages.)

Beans - Red beans, black beans, and kidney beans have all gained a reputation for being among the top ten foods that contain the highest levels of antioxidants. In addition, many beans have a high concentration of a substance known as beta-glucans, which has been shown to lessen the impact on blood sugar levels by lowering the pace at which carbs are digested. (If you have been eating a diet low in fiber, you should gradually increase the levels.)

Blueberries- Recent research has revealed that eating blueberries can help reduce inflammation. Blueberries are a good source of antioxidants.

Green tea is an excellent source of antioxidants due to its high catechin content. Green tea drinkers have been shown in many studies to have significantly lower levels of inflammation in their bodies than persons who don't drink it regularly. (A great antioxidant could be obtained from drinking three cups of strong green tea.)

Ginger- Ginger is an excellent treatment for high blood sugar levels and an effective approach to reducing inflammation. Ginger can also be used as an effective anti-inflammatory agent.

Olive oil- Is another fantastic anti-inflammatory food. It is one of the monounsaturated fats with therapeutic characteristics and is believed to assist in the battle against inflammation.

Papaya- It contains an enzyme known as papain, which is superior to those found in any other meal in its ability to digest and metabolize protein. Western pharmaceutical companies are increasingly incorporating papain into their products to reduce inflammation. It is important to note that papaya contains a lot of sugar. Ideally, it should be consumed a few times weekly to maintain stable blood sugar levels and reduce inflammation.

Red Wine- A powerful anti-inflammatory duo is formed when mixed with red wine and olive oil. Inflammation is halted dead in its tracks by the red wine, and olive oil seals the deal if there is any inflammation that manages to get through! (Those who can handle low levels of alcohol consumption should drink no more than one drink the size of a shot glass daily.)

Chapter Eight: Enhancing the Quality of Mealtimes

Anti-Inflammatory Cooking: A Gluten-Free (or Low Gluten Diet)

This gets down to the meat of the issue! Wheat consumption around the globe is at an all-time high. Everyone who experiences symptoms ranging from mild glucose intolerance to celiac disease can attest to this reality. For lunch and/or dinner, the typical American might eat toast, cereal, French toast, pancakes, pasta, pizza, or a sandwich. Wheat consumption in some form occurs three times a day in the diet of many households. Wheat may be consumed at every meal in a typical family, in addition to being consumed for snacks and sweets. The vast majority of the wheat we consume today has been subjected to extensive processing and refinement. A gluten concentration of around 90% can be found in wheat that has been genetically engineered.

Furthermore, it is quite probable that our body doesn't even recognize most of this wheat that has been unduly processed as appropriate food, which may lead to inflammation in the body. This reaction can initiate an allergic reaction, bring on the symptoms of arthritis, and promote disease and general bad health. In addition, citrus fruits have been shown to promote inflammation in the body; nevertheless, it is essential to remember that different people react in various ways to the same stimuli. Understanding how your body reacts to various foods, including gluten, can assist in determining an appropriate intake level for your family's requirements and health.

It is important to remember that even if you are aware of the foods that are the most beneficial for your health, you should still avoid eating excessive foods that have been overly processed, fried foods, and foods that contain hydrogenated oil. This is the case even if you know the foods most beneficial for your health. Foods that have undergone extensive processing are more likely to contain additives and preservatives, both of which place an unnecessary burden on the body due to the high levels of toxicity they contain and the fact that these foods have lost much of their nutritional value to maintain their shelf life.

The Anti-Inflammation Diet in Summary (Gluten-Free Version)

Learn to pay attention to your body's cues and remember that no set minimum or maximum amount of food must be consumed. Even if there is still food on your plate, you should stop eating when you reach a point where you feel pleasantly content. When you are hungry, you should never miss meals. Make an effort to incorporate the items indicated below and the appropriate portion quantities. And make sure you stick to a diet that consists of roughly 40% carbohydrates, 30% healthy fats, and 30% protein. Consume only foods that are grown organically whenever you can. Your meals and menu should be planned, and you should make an effort to avoid becoming fixated on any one kind of food. If you have opted to add gluten-free options to an anti-inflammatory diet, it is important to ensure that none of the products you buy contain gluten.

In addition to corn and rice, gluten-free grains include amaranth, millet, quinoa, sorghum, and teff.

Gluten-free food categories include

1. Grains: Eat one to two cups of cooked gluten-free grains daily to maintain weight. Available foods to eat under grains (all gluten-free) include amaranth, brown basmati (rice flour), buckwheat

(corn flour), millet, oatmeal, quinoa, spelt, sorghum, and teff. However, avoid products made with wheat, including bread, cereals, whole-wheat flour, white flour, and pasta.

2. Legumes: Feel free to submerse legumes in water overnight and simmer them the following day. Adzuki Beans (Pinto, Black, and Garbanzo Beans), Lentils, Kidneys, Fermented Soybeans, Mung Beans, and Split Peas are examples of food to eat under legumes. Notwithstanding, you should monitor tofu intake as it may cause an allergic reaction.

3. Seafood: You should choose wild fish instead of farmed fish when available. Eat three to four servings per week, baked, boiled, or poached. Deep sea and cold water choices provide an excellent source of fatty acids. Fish provide essential omega-3 fats. You can eat the following: Cod, Sardines, Haddock, Mackerel, Halibut, Trout, Tuna, Summer Flounder, and Wild Salmon. Avoid all shellfish (clams, crab, lobster, and shrimp)

4. Meat: Protein in all meals will help regulate blood sugar levels and maintain energy. You can eat Organic Turkey and Chicken, Free-range/organic Buffalo, Lamb and Meat (Organic), Wild Game, Venison, and Elk, but you should avoid Pork, all Beef that isn't organically raised. Stuck to limited amounts of free-range beef.

The Complete Anti-Inflammatory Diet for Beginners

5. Herbs and spices: You should not have any problems with selecting herbs and spices. Any herbs and spices are permissible.

6. Sweeteners: You should stick to very limited amounts of sweeteners. Brown Rice Syrup, Agave Syrup, Stevia, Pure Maple Syrup, and Raw Honey are safe to consume in very limited amounts. Keep in mind that absolutely no Nutra-Sweet or other sweetener is allowed. This includes all sugar.

7. Butter and Oil: One pound of organic butter can be mixed with a cup of 0.2 % olive oil and then stored as a buttery spread in the refrigerator. Use coconut oil for baking. For cooking, use olive oil. Organic Butter, in small amounts as a spread. For salads, use seed or nut oils.

8. Dairy Products and Eggs: Eat only organic eggs. Eating Commercial eggs or Dairy products (Yogurt, cheese, and cow milk) should be in moderation.

9. For miscellaneous, avoiding products made from corn, Fried foods, and Processed foods is to your benefit.

Emma Collins

Fast and Easy Gluten-Free Recipes

Because we live in a world that moves quickly and encourages eating on the go, our daily work and school schedules frequently do not give us sufficient time for us to shop for groceries, prepare meals, and eat calmly and collectedly. Our schedules frequently do not allow for regular meals or nutritious snacks to be consumed. It is not unheard of for people to eat at any time of the day, even before bed in the evening. Even though our digestive systems aren't operating at their peak levels while we sleep, we frequently subject them to one of the most taxing meals. Thanks to our eating habits, as much as 40 percent of our diet may consist of highly processed, pre-packaged meals.

A Seven-Day Meal Plan

Finding the right foods can pose additional problems for people who experience gluten sensitivity symptoms and allergies. Since, as we've learned, most processed foods contain gluten, we often have to search for those foods that are gluten-free. We often find ourselves asking, "Is this gluten-free?" Therefore, I have included gluten-free foods in the gluten-free diet plan. Hopefully, these simple meal ideas and gluten-free diet suggestions will help make your meal planning more relaxed and your meals more enjoyable! Organizing our gluten-free life and cutting our food bill with a gluten-free diet, I devised a way to simplify our lives while cutting our food bill. As a working couple, we recognize the value of our time and the ever-increasing cost of groceries for our families. One evening, shortly after we switched to a gluten-free diet, we discussed the number of hours we spent creating a gluten-free menu, shopping, and cooking for our family, only to start the whole process again.

I started making a list of menus and recipes. I have always found creative solutions to daily demands by making to-do lists and following through on tasks. You can say that is one of the perks of being a mother. I realized that my list could be an enjoyable and helpful tool for feeding my growing family a gluten-free diet while saving money! We also found that having a plan helps save money; it eliminates the late-afternoon frustration of deciding what to serve for dinner. My Strategy: I recycled the same recipes for most meals. So, I started by making a list of thirty gluten-free family favorites. Mostly, I included foods that our families preferred and easy and quick-to-prepare recipes. The recipes fell into a few categories: vegetarian, meat/chicken, salads/supper sandwiches, easy skillet and crock-pot meals, and pasta. I listed the main entrees in these categories until we reached 30 meals that each of our families especially enjoyed.

Another key consideration was the expense. Selecting less expensive ingredients substantially cut our food bill! Filling in the Blanks Next, I prepared a monthly calendar. At the top of each calendar square, I wrote down the meal I had designated for that day. I factored in-game/practice days, evening meetings, and dates when I expected guests. My goal was to include as many daily gluten-free meal requirements as possible. Below each main meal entry, I included side dishes that would add to our gluten-free meals. The final step was to create a gluten-free grocery list that could be used and reused. The beauty of this was that we could print out a new list each time we shopped and simply check what we needed to complete our meal requirements each month. Remember to include foods for breakfast, snacks, and lunch. You'll probably find there's a definite pattern to these meals. To create your four-week meal plan, follow these recommendations for the next two months and keep track of the changes! Final Thoughts. It may help to have two different gluten-free meal plans, one for winter and summer meals. It's also possible to remain flexible. If something unexpected comes up, simply swap out the meals. Photocopying pages from cookbooks may be helpful. Check out our eventual meal plan and a sample gluten-free list shopping in the next chapter, look forward to it!

Chapter Nine: Foods and Substitution

Sample Gluten-Free List – Shopping

Below is a gluten-free sample list for your shopping needs.

For gluten-free baking/cereals, you can get:

- Gluten-free grains
- Gluten-free rice
- Gluten-free oatmeal
- Gluten-free oats
- Gluten-free spaghetti
- Gluten-free macaroni

- Gluten-free Cornbread
- Gluten-free noodles
- Gluten-free Stuffing
- Gluten-free Cereals
- Gluten-free Granola
- Gluten-free pasta
- Gluten-free flour
- Gluten-free bread
- Gluten-free buns
- Gluten-free biscuits
- Gluten-free Rolls
- Gluten-free muffins
- Gluten-free wheat bread

For fruits and vegetables, here is a sample list:

- Bean sprouts, broccoli
- Red pepper
- Cabbage: red and green
- Leeks /onion
- Asparagus
- Rutabagas, turnips
- String beans
- Zucchini

The Complete Anti-Inflammatory Diet for Beginners

- Lettuce - green, mixed,
- Cantaloupe
- Melons
- Strawberries
- Rhubarb
- Citrus fruits, including oranges and grapefruit
- Bananas
- Apples
- Berries
- Peaches
- Pears

A sample gluten-free shopping list for dairy and eggs includes:

- Gluten-free cheese
- Gluten-free ice cream
- Gluten-free milk
- Organic eggs

For gluten-free snacks/desserts, you have:

- Gluten-free Crackers
- Gluten-free cupcakes
- Gluten-free brownies

A sample Gluten-free Drinks/Miscellaneous shopping list includes:

- Gluten-free drinks
- Gluten-free beer
- Gluten-free alcohol

For meats/poultry, here is a sample list:

- Gluten-free chicken
- Organic meats

For Soups/Sauces/Spreads/Condiments, you can have:

- Gluten-free soups
- Gluten-free sauces
- Gluten-free peanut butter
- Olive oil

What to eliminate, what to substitute, and the directions.

While eliminating butter, you can substitute it. Just:

- Blend organic butter and virgin olive oil (as a spread).

The Complete Anti-Inflammatory Diet for Beginners

- Blend organic butter and coconut oil (for baking).
- Non-hydrogenated vegan margarine

For these alternatives, equal quantities may be substituted.

To eliminate eggs, many people tolerate organic eggs. The following binders may also be substituted.

- Soaked Flaxseeds (overnight in water or boiled for 15 min. 1 to 2 tablespoons seeds in baked foods.
- Tofu is a great substitute for scrambled or baked goods by adding ½ to 1 cup of water.
- Banana binds baked goods (sweet) substitute by adding ¼ cup for 1 egg.
- Arrowroot powder (a binder for gluten-free flours) substitute by adding ½ to 1 banana for cookies or muffins.
- Guar gum (very small amount) substitute by adding 1 tablespoon for each cup of Gluten-free flour
- Xanthan gum substitute by adding ¼ to ½ teaspoon for baked goods

While eliminating chocolate, you can substitute with Carob powder – nutritionally better than chocolate! You can substitute 3 tablespoons for every ounce of chocolate for this alternative.

As you also eliminate cow's milk, substitute with Almond milk (or other nut milk), oat milk, rice milk, sesame seed milk, or soy milk. Equal quantities may be substituted.

Substitute peanut and peanut butter with almonds and almond butter. You may substitute with equal quantities.

Jerusalem artichokes, yucca root, and taro root are effective substitutes for potatoes and should be cooked similarly to potatoes.

Eliminate sugar and replace it with honey! Honey tends to be twice as sweet as processed cane sugar. You can substitute sugar with Pure Maple syrup, Brown rice syrup, or Stevia.

You could also eliminate wheat.

Note: When these flours are substituted, you may need to add slightly more baking soda or baking powder to increase rising. You can substitute with:

- Amaranth (usually has a strong flavor)
- Barley (small amount of gluten)
- Garbanzo Kamut (gluten)
- Oat (very small amounts of gluten)

- Quinoa (bitter, best when mixed with other flours)
- Rice (can be grainy; mix with other flours)
- Rye (contains gluten; should not be eaten every day)
- Soy (can have a beany flavor)
- Spelt (contains gluten; should not be eaten every day)

Modifying Recipes for an Anti-Inflammatory Gluten-Free Diet

Sample modified cookie recipe:

The following is a general guideline for adapting and changing recipes to fit anti-inflammatory diets and diets that do not contain gluten. I discovered that becoming accustomed to these adjustments required time and effort. Because the climate and the altitude make a difference, you must experiment differently. However, before you know it, you'll be able to whip up gourmet meals like a pro!

Recipe for the traditional "gluten-heavy" Fruit and Nut Cookies

6 cups of all-purpose flour
1 and a half cups of dark sugar

Emma Collins

1 and a half cups of white sugar

4 eggs

A cup and a half of butter

1 teaspoon salt

1 teaspoon baking soda

A couple of bags of chocolate chips

The quantities of sugar and flour that are called for need to be adjusted in the following way.

3 cups gluten-free flour in a measuring cup

1 and a half cups of honey

1 cup of organic butter 1 teaspoon of salt in the ocean

1 teaspoon aluminum-free baking soda

4 eggs from organic chickens (or 2 bananas mashed with 6 tablespoons of ground 51 flaxseeds rehydrated for 24 hours in a half cup of water.

2 cups of various nuts and/or seeds

1 cup of chopped fruit, including but not limited to apples and dates. Please take note that we have decreased the amount of butter by one-half and replaced the chocolate chips with seeds, fruit, and nuts in this recipe. Increase the butter in the recipe if you want the cookies to be flatter. These cookies are satisfying and aid in maintaining healthy blood sugar levels. This freshly baked cookie has some in it. Including just a little cinnamon

in your diet can assist in keeping the glucose level in check. There are a lot of fantastic options available for additional components!

Lists of Items to be kept on Hand Always

The following is a list of beneficial ingredients to keep on hand. You can add to y our list over time to avoid buying everything at once.

1. Almond butter
2. Beans and legumes, canned or dried
3. Brown rice, quinoa, oats, amaranth, and other grains
4. Brown rice syrup
5. Coconut oil (organic) for baking
6. Dried herbs and spices
7. Extra-virgin, cold-pressed olive oil
8. Filtered water
9. Fresh vegetables
10. Fresh fruits
11. Garlic
12. Gluten-free flour
13. Lemons
14. Milk substitutes such as rice milk, oat milk, soy milk, almond milk

15. Nuts and seeds
16. Onions
17. Rice, organic apple, balsamic, tarragon vinegars
18. Pure maple syrup
19. Raw honey and/or agave syrup
20. Large skillet or wok to stir-fry vegetables
21. Large pot for sauces and soups
22. Two-quart saucepan for cooking rice and other grains

Chapter Ten: Anti-inflammation Recipes & Meal Planning

The following chart shows a sample anti-inflammatory menu for one week. The program that I designed allows for meal flexibility. The anti-inflammation gluten-free diet is less of a diet than a healthy eating program. The beauty is that it can be adapted to suit the needs and dietary requirements of your family. I have deliberately not included specific food allotments for that reason. This book aims to help increase your awareness of the impact of diet on our lives. Whether you are searching for an anti-inflammatory diet, a gluten-free diet, or a combination of both, this book is designed just for you. The heart of the matter is to live a well-balanced life! Move more, drink the right amount of fresh, filtered water, and eat healthy fruits, vegetables, organic/homegrown eggs, poultry/meat, fresh cold water and farmed fish, dairy or soy products, and grains that are right for you. After four weeks of following this guide, your body will let you know!

Sample Anti-Inflammatory Menus for a Week

Below is a sample anti-inflammatory menu for a week:

Monday

On Monday, breakfast can be a 10-minute of Blueberry Oatmeal. Your morning snack can be Carob Chip Cookies. Lunch is a Gluten-Free Cream of Mushroom soup. The snack is Berry Medley Walnut Parfait with Coconut Vanilla Ice Cream. Dinner is Gluten-Free Teriyaki Salmon.

Tuesday

For Tuesday, breakfast is Egg Scramble. Morning snack Gluten-Free Almond Butter and Banana Sandwiches. Lunch is Hot Summer Chili. The snack is GF crackers and Peanut butter. Dinner is Honey Mustard Grilled Pork Chops.

The Complete Anti-Inflammatory Diet for Beginners

Wednesday

Breakfast on Wednesday will be Blueberry Buckwheat Pancakes. The morning snack will be Citrus Berry Parfait. Lunch is Salmon Egg Salad. Snack is GF Fruit ice cream, and dinner is Beef Stuffed Cabbage.

Thursday

For breakfast on Thursday, you will have Gluten-Free Banana Bread. For a morning snack, Gluten-Free Chocolate Cupcakes will do the trick. Lunch will be Fruity Chicken Salad. The snack will be GF Fruit ice cream, and the dinner will be Raw Veggie Nuts and Seeds Salad.

Friday

Friday will have you eating Gluten-Free Almond Raspberry Danish Tart for breakfast. The morning snack will be Garban Bean Chocolate Cake. Lunch will be Cedar Planked Salm Fillets. Snack will be a protein drink, and dinner will be Parmigi Beef Meatball.

Emma Collins

Anti-Inflammatory/Gluten-Free (Dinner) Menus for Four Weeks

First Week

Monday's dinner will be Spinach Mushroom Stuffed Chicken for the first week. Tuesday's will be Gluten-Free Teriyaki Salmon. Wednesday's will be Grilled Tilapia with Black Bean Mango Salsa. Thursday's will be Honey Mustard Grilled Pork Chops. Friday's will be Grilled Lemon Lime Cod Fillets.

Second Week

The second week will have you eating Raw Veggie Nuts and Seeds Salad for Monday's dinner, Lemon and Herb Crusted Salmon Fillets for Tuesday's dinner, Parmigiano Beef Meatballs for Wednesday's dinner, Spicy Almond Fish Sticks with Garlic Lime Tartar Sauce for Thursday's dinner and Grilled Rosemary Lime Swordfish for Friday's dinner.

Third Week

Monday's dinner will be Roasted Pork Tenderloin in the third week with Blueberry Sauce. Tuesday's dinner will be Gluten- Free Beef and Broccoli Stir-fry. Wednesday's dinner will be Spinach Mushroom Stuffed Chicken. Thursday's will be Beef Stuffed Cabbage, and Friday's will be Gluten- Free Teriyaki Salmon.

Fourth Week

The fourth week, Grilled Tilapia with Black Bean Mango Salsa, will be Monday's dinner. Raw Veggie Nuts and Seeds Salad for Tuesday's dinner, Gluten-Free Grilled Pineapple Burgers for Wednesday's dinner, Lemon and Herb Crusted Salmon Fillets for Thursday's dinner, and Honey-Mustard Lemon Marinated Chicken for Friday's dinner.

Emma Collins

Chapter Eleven: How to Cook and Prepare Food to Prevent Infection

Temperature control

In addition to the information presented here, all individuals involved in preparing and cooking food are required to read health and hygiene for food handlers. If you are sick with diarrhea or vomiting, you mustn't prepare or cook meals for others until you fully recover from your illness, as this can lead to infection, which will naturally lead to inflammation.

Purchasing edible products

If the site where you prepare the food is not close to your stores, you should put potentially dangerous foods that you buy into insulated bags or boxes so they may be transported safely.

Put any food that could make you sick into the refrigerator or the freezer as soon as possible.

Getting ready to cook the food

Make sure that your hands, clothes, and all of the equipment and the surfaces in the kitchen are clean before you start preparing the food. In addition, they will need to be kept clean during the entire food preparation process.

If your event will be conducted outside with few amenities, it is best to cook the food in a kitchen beforehand and then bring it to the event's location. This does not imply that the food needs to be cooked before it is brought to the gathering; nevertheless, preparations such as slicing raw meat so that it is ready to be cooked are required. Food made from scratch at the event and served immediately, like the food served at barbecues, have a lower risk of becoming contaminated than food cooked elsewhere and then transported to the event. As a result, you should aim to avoid pre-cooking food whenever it's possible and instead cook it at the event itself.

Preventing the food from becoming contaminated while it is being prepared.

Before beginning to prepare meals, it is imperative to remember to thoroughly clean and dry your hands. This is the single most critical step in the process.

When making food that will not be cooked before consumption, such as salads and sandwiches, it is important to use various equipment. You may find that wearing gloves is more comfortable; however, remember that each pair is intended for a specific purpose exclusively (for example, breaking up a cooked chicken for sandwiches). Put on a fresh pair of gloves before beginning the subsequent task.

Never use the same utensils for raw meats and foods that are ready to eat, such as cooked meats, unless those utensils have been thoroughly cleaned, sanitized, and dried. This helps prevent the spread of harmful bacteria. Don't forget bacterial infections can lead to inflammation.

Food that has been cooked and other foods that are ready to eat, such as salads, should always be served on clean and dry platters.

Cleaning and sanitizing utensils

To thoroughly clean and disinfect utensils, three steps must be followed in the proper order:

- Washing
- Sanitizing
- Drying.

It's important to give implements like cutting boards, bowls, and knives a thorough cleaning in water mixed with dish soap and warm water. When you're finished washing the utensils, they should have a clean appearance, and there shouldn't be any remnants of food or anything else visible. When cleaning is done properly, the vast majority of the potentially harmful bacteria will be removed. After that, the sterilization process will eliminate any that might have survived.

If a dishwasher has a hot wash cycle and a drying cycle, it can effectively clean and sanitize the dishes it washes. If you do not have access to a dishwasher, you will need to sanitize the items in a sink using either a chemical sanitizer or very hot water. Suppose you use a chemical sanitizer such as a sodium hypochlorite- or quaternary ammonium-based solution. In that case, you need to make sure that it is safe to use for sanitizing utensils that will be used for eating, drinking, and cooking. When using a certain sanitizer, paying close attention to the directions printed on the packaging is important. Take extra precautions to protect yourself from scalding if you use hot water.

After that, every utensil needs to be completely dried before it can be reused. If they are clean, tea towels can be used as an alternative to air drying, which is the preferred method.

If you are washing your hands at an event hosted outside, you should make sure that there is enough hot water available. If hot water is unavailable, it is recommended that disposable eating and drinking utensils be used and that sufficient cooking utensils be provided to last for the entirety of the event so that cleaning up after the event is not required.

Cooking

Always make sure the food is fully cooked. Preparing food only partially and then reheating it later is not safe. Chicken, sausages, and hamburgers should be cooked until the juices flow clear; however, the desired doneness of beef steaks can vary. If done correctly, cooking will lower potentially harmful germs to safe consumption levels. Keep in mind that some bacteria that cause food poisoning can resist cooking. Even though they will not be present in sufficient numbers to make someone sick immediately after the food is cooked, they can start growing again if the cooked food is left at temperatures between 5 and 60 degrees Celsius for an extended time. Because of this, prepared food must be cooled down as promptly as possible.

To the extent that it is feasible, you should attempt to cook food as close as possible to the time it will be served or sold. For instance, bring the food with you to the gathering and cook it there if you can do so. Because of this, there is a lower likelihood that the meal will become contaminated after it has been cooked. It also ensures that there won't be enough time for bacteria that cause food poisoning to develop to harmful levels in the food that has been prepared before it is consumed.

If it is not possible to cook food at the event, you will need to either pre-cook the food and transport it while it is still hot, or you can cook the meal, allow it to cool, and then transfer it while it is still cold.

Emma Collins

The process of chilling food

If you choose to pre-cook food before it cools, you will need to take extra precautions to ensure that the meal reaches a temperature of 5 degrees Celsius as quickly as possible. It may take up to twenty-four hours for a large container of cooked food stored in a refrigerator to chill to reach a temperature of five degrees Celsius. This is extremely risky because the interior of the meal will remain heated, which will encourage the growth of germs that cause food poisoning to hazardous levels.

According to the Food Safety Standards, food that has been cooked must be cooled to 5 degrees Celsius within six hours of being prepared. The temperature of the food must be lowered from 60 degrees Celsius to 21 degrees Celsius within two hours and then from 21 degrees Celsius to 5 degrees Celsius within a further four hours. It is possible to obtain safe cooling by:

- When the meal has been cooked, taking it from the top of the stove, the oven, or any other source of heat
- Allow the food to cool down outside the refrigerator, but ensure that it is stored inside the refrigerator as soon as any part of it reaches a temperature of 60 degrees Celsius or lower.
- Putting the food in containers with a small depth.

To ensure that the prepared meal is chilled within six hours, you will need to use your thermometer to monitor the cooling process.

Rewarming the food

Food brought to the event is cold but is supposed to be served hot will have to be heated up at the event until it is scalding hot in a hurry and then maintained at that temperature until it is served. It is recommended to reheat the food to a temperature of 70 degrees Celsius and then maintain it for a minimum of two minutes. Check, with the help of your thermometer, to see if all of the food has reached this temperature or higher.

Keeping food at a suitable temperature

At the event, hot food will need to be maintained at a temperature of at least 60 degrees Celsius. This could be accomplished by utilizing either gas or electric home appliances.

Emma Collins

Chapter Twelve: Money-Saving Tips for Preparing your Food

In these tough economic times, everyone is looking for ways to save money. One area where you can trim your budget is by preparing your food. Cooking at home is not only cheaper than eating out, but it can also be healthier and more satisfying. Here are some tips to help you save money on food:

Keep your Recipes Simple

When it comes to cooking, sometimes the simplest recipes are the best. Keep your recipes simple by using a few ingredients and taking shortcuts.

You'll still be able to make delicious, home-cooked meals without spending hours in the kitchen.

Here are some tips for keeping your recipes simple:

- Use fresh, seasonal ingredients whenever possible. Seasonal produce is generally cheaper and tastier than out-of-season options.

- Choose recipes with short ingredient lists. The fewer ingredients a recipe has, the less time it will take to make.

- Take shortcuts where you can. For example, use pre-chopped vegetables or canned broth instead of making everything from scratch.

By following these tips, you'll be able to make simple, delicious meals that your whole family will enjoy.

Make Swaps, Narrow It Down, or Leave It Out!

When it comes to cooking, there are always ways to make swaps, narrow them down, or leave them out. Here are some tips on how to do just that:

- When it comes to cooking, try to make swaps where you can. For instance, if a recipe calls for butter, you can try using olive oil instead. Or, if a recipe calls for white sugar, you can try using honey instead.

- If you're trying to narrow down a recipe, focus on the key ingredients. For instance, if you're making a soup, focus on vegetables and broth. You can always leave out the extras like croutons or cheese.

- And finally, if you're unsure about a recipe, or don't have all the ingredients on hand, don't be afraid to leave it out altogether!

Combine Similar Items

Whether you're trying to save money or time, cooking can be more efficient when you combine similar items. If you have a lot of vegetables that need to be used, consider making soup or stir-fry. These dishes are relatively quick and easy to make, allowing you to use various ingredients simultaneously.

If you have leftovers that need to be used up, think about how they could be incorporated into another meal. For example, leftover chicken can be shredded and added to a salad or wrapped in a tortilla for a quick and easy lunch. Get creative with your leftovers and see how many ways you can use them!

Finally, if you have any perishable items close to their expiration date, try to use them as soon as possible. This is especially important with meats and dairy products.

Make Your Meal Meatless

If you're looking to cut down on your meat consumption but don't want to sacrifice flavor or variety in your diet, try making some of your meals meatless. It can be easier to cook delicious, hearty meals without meat products. Plus, it's a great way to save money on your grocery bill.

Here are a few tips for making your meal meatless:

- Incorporate more vegetables into your diet. Vegetables are a great source of protein and can be used in place of meat in most recipes. Try substituting mushrooms, zucchini, or eggplant for ground beef in tacos or spaghetti sauce. You can also add extra veggies to soups and stews to make them more filling.

- Use beans or lentils as a protein source.

Better to cook at home than eat at a restaurant

It's no secret that cooking at home is cheaper than eating out. But in addition to saving money, cooking at home has other benefits. For one, you can control the quality and quantity of ingredients in your meals. You can also tailor your recipes to your specific dietary needs and preferences. And let's not forget the satisfaction of knowing you made a delicious meal from scratch!

If you're not confident in your cooking skills, plenty of resources are available to help you get started, including cookbooks, cooking classes, and online tutorials. With a bit of practice, you'll be whipping up healthy and affordable meals in no time. So next time you're tempted to order takeout, remember that cooking at home is better for your wallet and waistline. Also, don't forget if you need recipes to prepare your favorite dishes, there are very good examples included in this book.

How much does it cost to eat Gazpacho in a restaurant compared to cooking at home?

Many people love Gazpacho, but they might not realize how easy it is to cook at home. It's a great dish to make ahead of time and can be easily reheated or eaten cold. Plus, it's cheaper to make than eating out at a restaurant.

If you're wondering how much it would cost to eat Gazpacho in a restaurant, the average price is around $8-10 per dish. However, you can easily make Gazpacho at home for a fraction of the cost, which ranges between $3-5 per serving. You can check out the recipe for making a bowl of gazpacho in the recipes chapter.

So next time you're craving Gazpacho, why not try making it at home? It's cheaper and just as delicious!

Buy in Bulk

The holidays are a time for family, friends, and food. Lots and lots of food. Cooking for a crowd can be expensive, but there are ways to save money without skimping on quality or quantity. One way to do this is to buy in bulk.

Bulk buying is when you buy a large quantity of one item at a discount. This is usually only possible with non-perishable items like canned goods, dry goods, and paper products. However, it can also be done with fresh produce if you have the space to store it. Buying bulk can save you money in the long run, but it requires upfront planning and investment.

Plan Ahead

Planning your meals and recipes saves you money. It may seem daunting, but a little bit of planning can go a long way! Here are a few tips to get you started:

- Make a list of the recipes you want to make for the week. This will help you ensure you have all the ingredients and that you're not making too much food.

- Plan for leftovers! If you know you'll have extra food, save it for another meal. This will help reduce food waste and save you money in the long run.

- Use coupons and sales to your advantage. Keep an eye out for deals on ingredients that can be used in multiple recipes. This will help stretch your budget further.

Utilize your Freezer

Regarding cooking, your freezer is one appliance that can save you loads of money and time. Here are a few tips on how to make the most out of your freezer:

- Plan by cooking larger meals and portioning them into individual servings. This way, you'll always have a quick and easy meal when you're short on time or money.

- Make use of leftovers! Freeze them in individual portions so you can enjoy them later.

- Buy in bulk when groceries are on sale, and stock up your freezer. This way, you'll always have ingredients for your favorite recipes, saving money in the long run.

Emma Collins

Chapter Thirteen: What is Better for The Planet When it comes to food consumption

The foods we consume, however, are fueling some of the greatest dangers to the continued existence of humanity, which may seem like an ironic twist. According to a growing body of data, our current industrialized food production systems have been determined to be a contributor to climate change, a source of pollution, and a factor in the reduction of biodiversity.

Find out exactly what's in your food.

It is common practice to boost crop and livestock production by employing pesticides, herbicides, and antimicrobial medications; nevertheless, these practices frequently have unintended consequences for human health. In addition to polluting the land and aquatic environments, farm discharge can contaminate aquatic ecosystems.

Learn more about the origins of the foods you eat by perusing the labels, quizzing the manufacturer, and conducting online research. Whenever you have the option, choose whole foods from farms that practice sustainable agriculture rather than goods that come from intensive farms or are extensively processed. Instead of ordering takeout, you should cook your meals at home.

Start cultivating your garden.

When you grow your own food, you can avoid using harmful chemicals such as pesticides, unnecessary packaging and preservatives, and gasoline for transportation and cold chain storage. The most unaltered versions of fruits, vegetables, and herbs retain the highest levels of their respective nutrients. In addition to having anti-inflammatory and antioxidant properties, they are inexpensive and contain a high concentration of vitamins.

Build a community garden with your friends and neighbors by working together. You can cultivate edible plants in the area surrounding your house, on your balcony, or even on your windowsill.

Adopt a diet that is high in plant foods.

In recent years, there has been a significant increase in the demand for animal proteins that need a lot of resources. At the moment, over sixty percent of the world's agricultural land is used for the grazing of cattle, and people in many nations consume an unhealthy amount of food that is produced from animals.

Adopting diets high in plants would result in less land being used, less greenhouse gas being produced, less water required, and improved animal welfare. It would also make more cropland available, given that the global population is expected to reach 9 billion people by 2050. A shift toward diets that are higher in plant matter may also assist in lowering the incidence of chronic diseases, including heart disease, stroke, diabetes, and cancer, as well as the expenses of treatment and lost income connected with these conditions.

Diversify your diet

The diets of people all around the world are becoming more similar to one another, and a disproportionate amount of their food comes from crops that are high in energy but low in macronutrients. Over the past century, more than ninety percent of the world's crop varieties have vanished. Only nine different plant species are responsible for 66 percent of the world's crop production. Malnutrition affects up to one-third of the world's population, and many nations are simultaneously coping with the twin epidemics of undernutrition and overweight or obesity.

According to the findings of the EAT-Lancet Commission, switching to healthier diets that include a variety of plant-based foods and moving away from highly processed foods, as well as diets that are high in refined grain and added sugar, could prevent up to a quarter of all deaths that occur in adults.

Conclusion

A healthy future is within reach with the help of The Complete Anti-Inflammatory Diet for Beginners. This book provides readers with everything they need to know to make better choices for their health. This book is a comprehensive guide to healthier lifestyles, from grocery lists to recipes.

The anti-inflammatory diet is based on eating whole, unprocessed foods rich in nutrients. This way of eating has been shown to reduce inflammation throughout the body, leading to several health benefits. These benefits include weight loss, improved energy levels, and reduced risk of chronic diseases.

In a publication by the Harvard School of Public health, it was reported that a diet rich in vegetables and fruits could lower blood pressure, reduce the risk of heart disease and stroke, prevent some types of cancer, lower the risk of eye and digestive problems, and have a positive effect upon blood sugar, which can help keep appetite in check.

Ideally, following weeks of beginning a gluten-free diet, your symptoms should substantially improve. However, full recovery of your digestive system might take up to two years.

Going for an annual screening would be sufficient to provide you with a yearly evaluation during which your height, weight, and symptoms will be assessed.

It is recommended that a Mediterranean diet should follow a gluten and anti-inflammatory diet. This is because, according to Biomedical research by JW Thompson, Mediterranean Diet is rich in omega-3 fatty acids, an active nutrient found to be a good source of anti-inflammatory diets, so you should watch out for my next book.

The switch to an anti-inflammatory diet may seem daunting initially, but this book makes it easy. With clear instructions and delicious recipes, anyone can start living a healthier life today. So, what are you waiting for?

Emma Collins

Delicious Anti-Inflammation Recipes to Keep Your Family Healthy

Here are some recipes you can whip up for an anti-inflammatory diet.

Greek white beans in tomato sauce

INGREDIENTS

1 tablespoon extra-virgin olive oil

2 green onions, thinly sliced

2 large garlic cloves, minced

1 teaspoon tomato paste

2 x 400 g cans organic chopped tomatoes

1 teaspoon dried oregano

½ teaspoon smoked paprika (sweet)

Pinch chili flakes (optional)

1 bay leaf

2 x 400 g cans organic butter beans, drained and rinsed (alternatively fava beans)

sea salt and black pepper, to taste

2 large handfuls of baby spinach leaves (optional)

Flat leaf parsley to garnish

DIRECTIONS

1. Heat the oven to 350°F / 180°C.
2. Heat the oil in a large ovenproof skillet (I use a cast iron one) over medium heat. Then gently cook the onion and garlic with a pinch of salt for 8-10 minutes, until the onion is soft.
3. Stir in the tomato paste and cook for 1 minute, then add the tomatoes, oregano, paprika, bay leaf, chili flakes (if using), and butter beans. Season with freshly ground black pepper plus a pinch of salt. Increase heat to medium-high and bring to a light simmer. Note: depending on the brand of chopped tomatoes or how saucy I want the dish, I add 2-4 tablespoons of water to the pan before bringing it to a simmer.

4. Once the sauce starts to simmer, transfer it to the preheated oven for 25-30 minutes until thickened and bubbling.
5. Remove from the oven and stir in the baby spinach to wilt (about 1 minute).
6. Sprinkle with parsley (and crumbled feta, if desired) and serve as a main with some crusty bread as a side dish (served hot or cold).

Servings: 4

Spicy corn & black bean salad

INGREDIENTS

4 cups corn kernels
1 ½ tablespoons fajita seasoning
½ teaspoon ground black pepper
1 (15 ounce) can black beans, drained and rinsed
1 red bell pepper, chopped
½ cup chopped green onion
¼ cup chopped fresh cilantro
¼ cup fresh lime juice
2 tablespoons orange juice

DIRECTIONS

1. Heat olive oil in a large skillet over medium heat. Cook and stir corn, fajita seasoning, and black pepper in the hot oil until corn is lightly browned 6 to 8 minutes. Remove from heat and set aside to cool.
2. Mix corn mixture, black beans, red bell pepper, green onion, jalapeno pepper, cilantro, lime juice, orange juice, and salt

Emma Collins

together in a bowl; cover and refrigerate for at least 1 hour before serving.

Servings: 8

Hummus with veggies

INGREDIENTS

¾ cup mixed vegetables, such as baby carrots, cherry tomatoes, and red bell pepper slices

3 tablespoons prepared hummus

DIRECTIONS

1. Wash vegetables and slice them into bite sizes
2. Arrange them on a platter
3. Dip vegetables into hummus

Servings: 1

Emma Collins

Vegetarian chili

INGREDIENTS

2 tablespoons extra-virgin olive oil
1 medium yellow onion, diced medium
4 garlic cloves, roughly chopped
1 ½ teaspoons ground cumin
1 teaspoon chipotle chili powder
Coarse salt and ground pepper
1 medium zucchini, cut into ½-inch dice
¾ cup (6 ounces) tomato paste
1 can (15.5 ounces) of black beans, rinsed and drained
1 can (15.5 ounces) of pinto beans, rinsed and drained
1 can (14.5 ounces) diced tomatoes with green chiles
1 can (14.5 ounces) of diced tomatoes

DIRECTIONS

1. In a large pot, heat oil over medium-high. Add onion and garlic; frequently cook until onion is translucent and garlic is soft about 4 minutes.

2. Add cumin and chili powder, season with salt and pepper, and cook until spices are fragrant for 1 minute.
3. Add zucchini and tomato paste; frequently cook until the paste is deep brick red for 3 minutes.
4. Stir in black beans, pinto beans, and cans of diced tomatoes.
5. Add 2 cups of water and bring the mixture to a boil. Reduce to a medium simmer and cook until zucchini is tender and liquid reduced slightly by 20 minutes.
6. Season with salt and pepper.

Servings: 4 to 6

Emma Collins

Creamy polenta with ratatouille

INGREDIENTS

Olive Oil

1 medium onion, diced

several sprigs of fresh oregano or marjoram (or 1 teaspoon dried)

1 sprig of fresh rosemary (or ½ teaspoon dried)

2-3 garlic cloves, minced

4 cups eggplant peeled and cubed

2 cups diced pepper (red, orange, yellow, or green)

4 cups peeled and seeded tomatoes, chopped

½ teaspoon dried turmeric

1 bay leaf

a handful of fresh basil, chopped

1 pack instant polenta

DIRECTIONS

1. Assemble all ingredients
2. Prepare the eggplant: peel and cube, place in a colander
3. Sprinkle with salt and drain for 15-20 minutes while you chop and measure the other ingredients.

4. This is not an essential step, but it releases excess water from the eggplant, making it firmer and meatier.
5. Heat a large skillet over medium-high heat. When hot, add 1-2 tablespoons olive oil and sauté the onions for 5-6 minutes until they start to brown on the edges.
6. Add garlic and continue to sauté for another minute.
7. Add eggplant and peppers, and cook until they just begin to soften.
8. Add remaining ingredients, except the basil, stir gently, cover, and reduce heat to a simmer.
9. Cook for 20-25 minutes until vegetables are tender and flavors have come together.
10. Add fresh chopped basil and combine – ready to serve
11. Cook polenta until soft
12. Add more liquid to make it creamier
13. Add grated parmesan
14. Serve ratatouille over polenta with extra basil and parmesan.

Servings: 4

Emma Collins

Baked Oatmeal

INGREDIENTS

2 cups/7 Ounce rolled oats

½ cup/2 Ounce walnut pieces, toasted and chopped

1/3 cup/2 Ounce natural cane sugar or maple syrup, plus more for serving

1 teaspoon aluminum-free baking powder

1 ½ teaspoons ground cinnamon

Scant ½ teaspoon fine-grain sea salt

2 cups/475 ml milk

1 large egg

3 tablespoons unsalted butter, melted and cooled slightly

2 teaspoons pure vanilla extract

2 ripe bananas, cut into 1/2-inch/1 cm pieces

1 ½ cups/6.5 Ounce huckleberries, blueberries, or mixed berries

DIRECTIONS

1. Preheat the oven to 375°F/190°C with a rack in the top third of the oven. Generously butter the inside of an 8-inch/20cm square baking dish.

2. Mix the oats, half the walnuts, and the sugar in a bowl, if using the baking powder, cinnamon, and salt.
3. In another bowl, whisk together the maple syrup, if using the milk, egg, half of the butter, and vanilla.
4. Arrange the bananas in a single layer at the bottom of the prepared baking dish.
5. Sprinkle two-thirds of the berries over the top.
6. Cover the fruit with the oat mixture.
7. Slowly drizzle the milk mixture over the oats. Gently give the baking dish a few thwacks on the countertop to ensure the milk moves through the oats. Scatter the remaining berries and remaining walnuts across the top.
8. Bake for 35 to 45 minutes, until the top, is golden and the oat mixture has set.
9. Remove from the oven and let cool for a few minutes.
10. Drizzle the remaining melted butter on the top and serve.
11. Sprinkle with more sugar or drizzle with maple syrup if you want it sweeter.

Servings: 6

Emma Collins

Breakfast casserole

INGREDIENTS

Nonstick cooking spray

1 pound ground maple pork sausage

6 slices of soft hearty white bread

One 8-ounce package of shredded triple cheddar cheese

8 large eggs

2 cups whole milk

1 teaspoon dry mustard

¼ teaspoon salt

½ teaspoon seasoned pepper

DIRECTIONS

1. Preheat the oven to 350°F / 167°C. Spray a 13-by-9-inch baking sheet with nonstick cooking spray.
2. In a large skillet, cook the sausage over medium heat, stirring, until brown and crumbly, about 10 minutes; drain well on paper.
3. Cut and discard the crust of the bread. Cut the slices in half, and arrange them in a single layer in the prepared baking dish, cutting

pieces to fit as necessary to cover the bottom of the dish. Sprinkle with the sausage and cheese.
4. In a large bowl, whisk together the eggs, milk, mustard, seasoned, and pepper; carefully pour the mixture over the cheese.
5. Bake the casserole until set and golden, about 40 minutes.
6. Let stand for 10 minutes before serving.

Servings: 8 to 10

Emma Collins

Felafel with tahini & tzatziki

INGREDIENTS

For the Tzatziki
7 ounces of Greek Yogurt
½ cup peeled and diced seedless cucumber
1 tablespoon lemon juice
1 garlic clove
½ teaspoon salt
¼ teaspoon dried mint
Pinch of black pepper

For the Tahini Sauce
1/3 cup tahini paste
½ lemon juice
3 tablespoons water
salt and pepper to taste
For the Falafel Burgers:
2 cans chickpeas, drained
1 small red onion
3 tablespoons flour
4 cloves garlic

1 tablespoon cumin

1 tablespoon chili powder

1 tablespoon coriander

1 teaspoon turmeric

1 teaspoon salt

3-4 tablespoons olive oil, divided

4 Rolls

Tomatoes

sliced cucumber

Other toppings ideas: Lettuce, Red Onion, Feta, Kalamata Olives

DIRECTIONS

For the Tzatziki

1. Mix all ingredients and set aside.

For the Tahini Sauce

1. Mix all ingredients and set aside.

For the Falafel Burgers

Emma Collins

1. Add the chickpeas, onion, garlic, flour, and spices (cumin, chili powder, coriander, turmeric, and salt) into the food processor and pulse until combined (add additional flour until it holds together).
2. Divide the mixture into equal-sized patties
3. Heat 1-2 tablespoons of olive oil in a large nonstick skillet over medium-high heat.
4. Add two falafel patties to the preheated skillet and cook for 4 minutes.
5. Gently flip patties (they are fragile!) and cook for an additional 4 minutes.
6. Remove from the skillet and set aside (either keep in a warm oven or under some aluminum foil).
7. Add the remaining olive oil and repeat the process with the remaining 2 patties.
8. To serve: toast up buns for a few minutes under the broiler. Spread some tahini sauce on the bottom bun and top with a falafel patty. Top with desired toppings, followed by a dollop of tzatziki. Serve while hot!

Servings: 4

Gazpacho

INGREDIENTS

1 hothouse cucumber, halved and seeded, but not peeled
2 red bell peppers, cored and seeded
4 plum tomatoes
1 red onion
2 garlic cloves, minced
23 ounces tomato juice (3 cups)
¼ cup white wine vinegar
¼ cup good olive oil
½ tablespoon kosher salt
1 teaspoon freshly ground black pepper

DIRECTIONS

1. Roughly chop the cucumbers, bell peppers, tomatoes, and red onions into 1-inch cubes.
2. Put each vegetable separately into a food processor fitted with a steel blade and pulse until it is coarsely chopped. Do not overprocess!

3. After each vegetable is processed, combine them in a large bowl and add the garlic, tomato juice, vinegar, olive oil, salt, and pepper.
4. Mix well and chill before serving.
5. The longer the gazpacho sits, the more the flavors develop.

Servings: 4-6

Roasted Garlic Cauliflower Soup

INGREDIENTS

1 large head cauliflower (about 2 ½ lb.)
4 ½ teaspoons olive oil
1 ½ teaspoons kosher salt, divided
3 garlic cloves, unpeeled
3 cups reduced-sodium chicken broth
1 cup 2% reduced-fat milk
½ cup grated Manchego or Parmesan cheese
Freshly ground black pepper
Garnishes: olive oil, pomegranate seeds, fresh thyme leaves

DIRECTIONS

1. Preheat the oven to 425°F/218°C. Cut cauliflower into 2-inch florets; toss with olive oil and 1/2 tsp. Salt. Arrange florets in a single layer on a jelly-roll pan. Wrap garlic cloves in aluminum foil and place on a jelly-roll pan with the cauliflower.
2. Bake at 425°F/218°C for 30 to 40 minutes or until cauliflower is golden brown, tossing cauliflower every 15 minutes.

3. Transfer cauliflower to a large Dutch oven. Unwrap garlic, and cool for 5 minutes. Peel garlic and add to cauliflower. Add stock and bring to a simmer over medium heat; simmer, occasionally stirring, for 5 minutes. Let the mixture cool for 10 minutes.
4. Process cauliflower mixture, in batches, in a blender until smooth, stopping to scrape down sides as needed.
5. Return cauliflower mixture to Dutch oven; stir in milk, cheese, and 1 tsp. Salt. Cook over low heat, occasionally stirring, for 2 to 3 minutes or until thoroughly heated. Add pepper to taste.

Servings: 6 to 8

Bean Burger

INGREDIENTS

2 cans (15.5 ounces each) of black, white, or pinto beans or black-eyed peas
1 cup dried breadcrumbs
2 large eggs, lightly beaten
1 teaspoon coarsely ground black pepper
½ teaspoon garlic powder
Extra Flavorings (see Burger options)
6 good-quality hamburger buns

DIRECTIONS

1. Drain 1 can of beans, reserving the liquid, and mash the beans in a medium bowl.
2. Drain the second can, and add to the bowl with the breadcrumbs, eggs, pepper, and garlic powder.
3. Stir in Extra Flavorings if using. If necessary, add a little of the bean liquid until the mixture holds together but is not wet.
4. Divide into 6 equal portions and shape into 4-inch patties.
5. Warm the buns in a 300°F/149°C oven for about 5 minutes.

6. Meanwhile, heat ⅔ cup olive or canola oil in a large (12-inch) skillet over medium-high heat.
7. Add the patties and cook, turning only once, until a crisp brown crust forms on both sides, about 6 minutes total.
8. If you've chosen a burger that gets topped with cheese, add it now. Cover the skillet, turn the heat to low, and let the burgers continue to cook until the cheese melts. Top the burgers as desired.

Servings: 6

Frittata with low-fat cheese

INGREDIENTS

8 eggs
2 tablespoons finely chopped fresh oregano
½ teaspoon salt
¼ teaspoon freshly ground pepper
2 tablespoons extra-virgin olive oil
1 cup sliced red bell pepper
1 bunch of scallions, trimmed and sliced
½ cup crumbled goat cheese

DIRECTIONS

1. Position the rack in the upper third of the oven; preheat the broiler.
2. Whisk eggs, oregano, salt, and pepper in a medium bowl. Heat oil in a large, ovenproof, nonstick skillet over medium heat. Add bell pepper and scallions and cook, constantly stirring, until the scallions are just wilted, 30 seconds to 1 minute.
3. Pour the egg mixture over the vegetables and cook, lifting the edges of the frittata to allow the uncooked egg to flow underneath

until the bottom is light golden, 2 to 3 minutes. Dot the top of the frittata with cheese, transfer the pan to the oven, and broil until puffy and lightly golden on top, 2 to 3 minutes. Let rest for about 3 minutes before serving.
4. Serve hot or cold!

Servings: 4 to 6

Polenta lasagna

INGREDIENTS

1 (26-ounce) jar marinara sauce, divided
1 teaspoon olive oil
1 cup finely chopped onion
½ cup chopped red bell pepper
1 cup meatless fat-free sausage, crumbled (such as Lightlife Gimme Lean)
1 cup chopped mushrooms
½ cup chopped zucchini
2 garlic cloves, minced
1 (16-ounce) tube of polenta, cut into 18 slices
½ cup (2 ounces)

Emma Collins

Shredded part-skim mozzarella cheese

DIRECTIONS

1. Preheat the oven to 350°F/180°C.
2. Spoon ½ cup marinara sauce into an 8-inch square baking dish to cover the bottom, and set aside. Heat oil in a large nonstick skillet over medium-high heat. Add onion and bell pepper; sauté for 4 minutes or until tender. Stir in sausage; cook for 2 minutes.
3. Add mushrooms, zucchini, and garlic; sauté for 2 minutes or until mushrooms are tender, stirring frequently. Add remaining marinara sauce; reduce heat, and simmer for 10 minutes.
4. Arrange 9 polenta slices over marinara in a baking dish, and top evenly with half of the vegetable mixture. Sprinkle ¼ cup of cheese over the vegetable mixture; arrange the remaining polenta over the cheese. Top polenta with the remaining vegetable mixture, and sprinkle with the remaining ¼ cup cheese.
5. Cover and bake at 350°F/180°C for 30 minutes. Uncover and bake for an additional 15 minutes or until bubbly. Let stand 5 minutes before serving.

Servings: 6

Lentil burger

INGREDIENTS

1 large clove of garlic, peeled
¼ teaspoon kosher salt
½ cup walnuts, toasted
2 slices of whole-wheat sandwich bread, crusts removed, torn into pieces
1 tablespoon chopped fresh marjoram or 1 teaspoon dried
¼ teaspoon freshly ground pepper
1 ½ cups cooked or canned (rinsed) lentils
2 teaspoons Worcestershire sauce, vegetarian or regular
3 teaspoons canola oil, divided
4 whole-wheat hamburger buns, toasted
4 pieces of leaf lettuce
4 slices tomato or jarred roasted red pepper
4 thin slices of red onion

DIRECTIONS

1. Coarsely chop the garlic; sprinkle with salt, and mash to a paste with the side of the knife. Coarsely chop walnuts in a food processor.

2. Add bread, marjoram, pepper, and garlic paste; process until coarse crumbs form.
3. Add lentils and Worcestershire; process until the mixture just comes together in a mass. Form into four 3-inch patties (about 1/3 cup each).
4. Heat 2 teaspoons of oil in a large nonstick skillet over medium heat. Cook the patties until browned on the bottom, 2 to 4 minutes.
5. Carefully turn over; reduce heat to medium-low. Drizzle the remaining 1 teaspoon of oil around the burgers and cook until browned on the other side and heated through for 4 to 6 minutes more.
6. Serve on buns with lettuce, tomato (or red pepper), and onion.

Servings: 4

Lentil Meatloaf

INGREDIENTS

Loaf

1 cup dry lentils (use green/brown)

2 ½ cups water or vegetable broth

3 tablespoons flaxseed meal (ground flaxseeds)

1/3 cup water (6 tablespoons)

2 tablespoons olive oil for sauteing or steam sauté using ¼ cup water

3 garlic cloves, minced

1 small onion, finely diced

1 small red bell pepper, finely diced

1 carrot, finely diced or grated

1 celery stalk, finely diced

¾ cup oats (I used Gluten Free oats)

½ cup oat flour or finely ground oats (any flour of choice will work here too)

1 heaping teaspoon of dried thyme

½ heaping teaspoon of cumin

½ teaspoon each garlic powder & onion powder…for good measure!

¼ – ½ teaspoon ground chipotle pepper, optional cracked pepper & sea salt to taste

Emma Collins

Glaze

3 tablespoons organic ketchup

1 tablespoon balsamic vinegar

1 tablespoon pure maple syrup

DIRECTIONS

1. Rinse lentils. In a large pot, add 2 ½ cups of water with lentils. Bring to a boil, reduce heat, cover, and simmer for about 40 minutes, stirring occasionally. It's ok if they get mushy; we are going to puree ¾ roughly of the mixture when cooled. Once done, remove the lid and set it aside to cool (do not drain). They will thicken a bit upon standing; about 15 minutes is good.
2. Preheat the oven to 350°F/180°C.
3. In a small bowl, combine a flaxseed meal and 1/3 cup water, and set aside for at least 10 minutes, preferably in the refrigerator. This will act as a binder and will thicken nicely upon sitting.
4. Prepare vegetables. In a sauté pan, heat oil or water over medium heat. Sauté garlic, onion, bell pepper, carrots, and celery for about 5 minutes. Add spices mixing well to incorporate. Set aside to cool.
5. Using an immersion blender or food processor, blend ¾ of the lentil mixture. For me, this was an important part, I tried it other ways, and this worked to help as a binder. If using an immersion

blender, tilt your pot slightly to the side for easier blending. Alternatively, you can mash the lentils with a potato masher or fork.
6. Combine sauteed vegetables with lentils, oats, oat flour, and flax egg, and mix well. Taste, add salt and pepper as needed, or any other herb or spice you like. Place the mixture into a loaf pan lined with parchment paper, leaving it overlapping for easy removal later. Press down firmly, filling in along the edges too.
7. Prepare your glaze by combining all ingredients in a small bowl and mixing until incorporated. I recommend making each tablespoon heaping, so you have plenty of this great sauce. Spread over the top of the loaf and bake in the oven for about 45 – 50 minutes. Let cool a bit before slicing.

Servings: 8

Emma Collins

Broccoli Souffle

INGREDIENTS

3 cups frozen chopped broccoli, thawed and drained
2 tablespoons butter
2 tablespoons all-purpose flour
½ teaspoon salt
½ cup milk
¼ cup grated Parmesan cheese

DIRECTIONS

1. In a saucepan over medium heat, cook and stir broccoli and butter until the butter is melted. Set 2 tablespoons broccoli aside for topping. Add flour and salt to the remaining broccoli; stir until blended. Gradually add milk. Bring to a boil; cook and stir for 2 minutes or until thickened. Remove from the heat; add cheese, stirring until cheese is melted.
2. In a large bowl, beat egg yolks until thickened and lemon-colored, about 5 minutes. Add broccoli mixture and set aside. In a small bowl, beat egg whites until stiff peaks form; fold into broccoli mixture.

3. Pour into an ungreased 1-½-qt. Deep round baking dish. Bake uncovered at 350°F/180°C for 20 minutes. Sprinkle with the reserved broccoli. Bake 10 minutes longer or until a knife inserted near the center comes out clean.

Servings: 2

Emma Collins

Veggie Terrines

INGREDIENTS

Kosher salt
8 large beet greens or ruby Swiss chard
Butter, softened, for greasing the mold
4 ounces cauliflower florets
4 ounces carrots
4 ounces green peas
1 red pepper
2 ¼ cups/560 ml heavy cream
5 eggs
1 ½ ounces/1/3 cup grated Parmesan cheese
Freshly ground black pepper

DIRECTIONS

1. Bring a large pot of water to a boil. Salt it and blanch the beet greens for 1 minute. Remove the leaves and immediately rinse them under ice-cold water to set their color. Gently lay flat on tea towels and pat dry with another tea towel. They should be completely dry.

2. Line a buttered terrine mold with a piece of parchment. Neatly lay in the beet leaves to cover the bottom and sides completely. They should dangle over the sides a bit so they can be folded over the completed terrine later.
3. Cook the cauliflower, carrots, and peas one at a time in the same pot of boiling salted water until very tender.
4. Remove them and immediately rinse them in ice-cold water to preserve their color. Drain well. Roast the pepper until very soft. Peel, seed, and cut into pieces.
5. Heat the oven to 350°F/180°C.

Servings: 8

Emma Collins

Jamaican Rice and Peas

INGREDIENTS

1 can (19 Ounce) of Kidney beans, including liquid
1 can (14 Ounce) Coconut milk
Water (approx. 1-2/3 cups)
2 cloves Garlic, chopped
1 Small onion or 2 stalks of scallion, chopped
1 tsp Dried thyme
1½ to 2 tsp Salt, to taste
3 tsp margarine (optional)
1 tsp Black Pepper
2 cups long-grain rice (rinsed and drained)

DIRECTIONS

1. Drain the liquid from the can of beans into a measuring cup and add the can of coconut milk and enough water to make four cups of liquid
2. Add liquid, beans, garlic, chopped onion, and thyme to a large pot
3. Add salt and black pepper. Bring to a boil.
4. Add rice and boil on High for 2 minutes.

5. Turn heat to Low and cook covered until all water is absorbed (about 15 to 20 min).
6. Fluff with a fork before serving.

Servings: 6 to 8

Emma Collins

Pomegranate Smoothie

INGREDIENTS

½ cup chilled pomegranate juice
½ cup vanilla low-fat yogurt
1 cup frozen mixed berries

DIRECTIONS

1. Add the juice, yogurt, and berries to a blender. Cover and blend until pureed

Servings: One 8-ounce serving

Watermelon-Pineapple-Ginger Juice

INGREDIENTS:

1/3 pineapple, cored and skin removed
2 large watermelon slices
1 inch (2.5 cm) piece of fresh ginger root

DIRECTIONS

1. Cut pineapple away from the core and rind.
2. Wash the watermelon well and cut 2 large slices. You can juice the rind as well as the flesh of the watermelon.
3. Wash ginger root and cut a 1 in (2.5 cm) piece to juice.
4. Place all ingredients into the juicer.
5. Juice.
6. Pour over ice and enjoy!

Servings: 1

Emma Collins

Rice with vermicelli

INGREDIENTS

4 tbsp. butter
½ cup thin vermicelli, broken into small pieces
1 cup rice, rinsed
2¼ cups boiling water
¾ tsp. Salt
¼ tsp. Pepper
¼ tsp. cinnamon

DIRECTIONS

1. In a frying pan, melt butter, then sauté vermicelli over medium/low heat, stirring until the pieces just begin to turn golden brown.
2. Add rice; stir-fry for a further 1 minute. Stir in the remaining ingredients, except for cinnamon, then bring to a boil.
3. Cover and cook over low heat for 12 minutes. Turn off the heat; stir. Recover and allow to cook in own steam for 30 minutes.
4. Place on a platter, lightly sprinkle with cinnamon and serve as a side dish with vegetable stew entrees.

The Complete Anti-Inflammatory Diet for Beginners

Servings: 3

Emma Collins

Warm Eggplant and Goat Cheese Sandwiches

INGREDIENTS

1 teaspoon olive oil

2 (¼-inch) vertical slices of small eggplant

Cooking spray

¼ teaspoon salt

¼ teaspoon freshly ground black pepper

¼ cup (2 ounces) goat cheese, softened

2 (1 ½-ounce) rustic sandwich rolls

2 (¼-inch) slices of tomato

1 cup arugula

DIRECTIONS

1. Preheat the oven to 275°F/135°C.
2. Brush oil over the eggplant.
3. Heat a large nonstick skillet coated with cooking spray over medium-high heat. Add eggplant; cook for 5 minutes on each side or until lightly browned. Sprinkle with salt and pepper.

4. Spread about 1 tablespoon of goat cheese over half the cut side of each roll. Place rolls on a baking sheet, cheese sides up; bake at 275°F/135°C for 8 to 10 minutes or until thoroughly heated.
5. Remove the top and bottom half of each roll from the oven with 1 eggplant slice, 1 tomato slice, and ½ cup arugula. Top sandwiches with the top halves of rolls.

Servings: 1

Emma Collins

Tomato crostini

INGREDIENTS

½ cup chopped plum tomato

1 tablespoon chopped fresh basil

1 tablespoon chopped pitted green olives

1 teaspoon capers

½ teaspoon balsamic vinegar

½ teaspoon olive oil

⅛ teaspoon sea salt

Dash of freshly ground black pepper

1 garlic clove, minced

4 (1-inch-thick) slices of French bread baguette

Cooking spray

1 garlic clove, halved

DIRECTIONS

1. Preheat the oven to 375°F/135°C.
2. Combine the first 9 ingredients.

3. Lightly coat both sides of the bread slices with cooking spray; arrange the bread slices in a single layer on a baking sheet. Bake at 375°F for 4 minutes on each side or until lightly toasted.
4. Rub 1 side of bread slices with halved garlic; top evenly with tomato mixture.

Servings: 1

Emma Collins

Lemon and roasted sage chicken

INGREDIENTS

2 lemons, thinly sliced
6 fresh sage leaves
1 (6-pound) chicken
3 teaspoons olive oil, divided
¾ pound parsnips, peeled and trimmed
¾ pound carrots, peeled and trimmed
½ pound turnips, peeled and trimmed
1 pound fingerling potatoes, halved
2 tablespoons chopped fresh thyme

DIRECTIONS

1. Preheat the oven to 425°F/218°C. Place 6 lemon slices and sage leaves under the skin of the chicken. Put the remaining lemon into the cavity. Tie legs together with twine, and tuck wings under. Brush 1 teaspoon of oil over the chicken. Place chicken in a roasting pan; roast in the lower third of the oven for 1 hour 15 minutes or until an instant-read thermometer registers

165°F/74°C. Transfer chicken to a cutting board; let rest for 15 minutes.
2. Meanwhile, cut root vegetables into matchsticks. Toss with potatoes in a baking pan with the remaining oil and thyme. Roast, stirring occasionally, for 45 minutes or until tender.
3. Remove skin from chicken. Discard lemons from the cavity. Slice enough chicken to serve 4 (such as breasts) and serve with half of the vegetables.

Servings: 5

Emma Collins

Orange and Duck Confit Salad

INGREDIENTS

1 tablespoon sherry vinegar

4 blood oranges, divided (3 sectioned, about 1 cup; 1 juiced, about ¼ cup)

1 teaspoon Dijon mustard

1 tablespoon olive oil

¼ teaspoon salt

¼ teaspoon pepper

1 small duck confit leg (5-6 ounces), shredded skin, fat, and bones discarded (about ¾ cup)

6 cups mixed winter salad greens (such as romaine, escarole, and spinach)

¼ cup skinned chopped hazelnuts, toasted

DIRECTIONS

1. In a small bowl, combine vinegar, orange juice, mustard, and oil, whisking well. Whisk in salt and pepper.
2. Combine shredded duck, salad greens, hazelnuts, and orange sections in a large bowl. Drizzle with vinaigrette; serve.

Servings: 4

Emma Collins

Zucchini Spaghetti

INGREDIENTS

3 Zucchini (cut to resemble spaghetti)
1 ½ cups Arugula
1 ½ cups Basil Leaves
1/3 cup Walnuts
2 Garlic Cloves (smashed)
½ cup Grated Parmesan Cheese
Olive Oil
Salt
Freshly Cracked Black Pepper
Coarse Homemade Breadcrumbs (toasted to garnish)

DIRECTIONS

1. Place the Arugula, Basil, Walnuts, Garlic, and Cheese in a food processor and begin to pulse. Slowly drizzle in Olive Oil and pulse until the mixture resembles a coarse paste. Season with Salt and Pepper to taste.
2. Heat a large skillet over medium-high with a few tablespoons of Olive Oil. Add the Zucchini and toss to coat in Oil.

3. Add a few tablespoons of Pesto and toss with the Zucchini. Once the Zucchini begins to take on color, transfer to a platter and top it with the toasted Breadcrumbs to taste.
4. Serve warm or at room temperature.
5. You may cut the Zucchini with a spiralizer, a mandolin fitted with a julienne attachment, or shave thinly with a peeler.

Servings: 4

Made in United States
North Haven, CT
21 November 2023